CHOLESTEROL LOWERING THERAPIES AND DRUGS

Edited by **Chunfa Huang** and **Carl Freter**

Cholesterol Lowering Therapies and Drugs
http://dx.doi.org/10.5772/61647
Edited by Chunfa Huang and Carl Freter

Contributors
Min-Ji Charng, Gamaleldin Ibrahim Harisa, Sabry Attia, Nduna Dzimiri, Maha M. Alrasheed, Alexander Orekhov, Ekaterina Ivanova, Marek Kučera, Ph.D., MsC., Stanislav Oravec, Ludovit Gaspar, Zaid Almarzooq, Parmanand Singh, Chunfa Huang

Published by InTech
Janeza Trdine 9, 51000 Rijeka, Croatia

Publishing Process Manager Edi Lipovic
Technical Editor SPi Global
Cover InTech Design team

First published October, 2016
Printed in Croatia

Additional hard copies can be obtained from orders@intechopen.com

Cholesterol Lowering Therapies and Drugs, Edited by Chunfa Huang and Carl Freter
p. cm.
Print ISBN 978-953-51-2734-5
Online ISBN 978-953-51-2735-2

For EU product safety concerns:
IN TECH d.o.o., Prolaz Marije Krucifikse Kozulić 3, 51000 Rijeka, Croatia,
info@intechopen.com or visit our website at intechopen.com.

Meet the editors

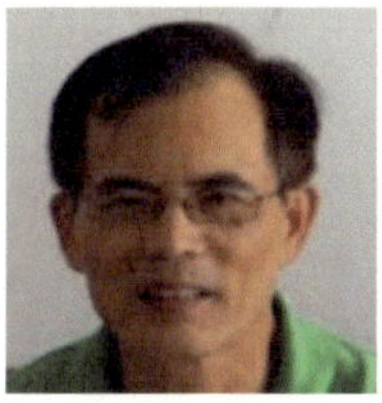

Dr. Chunfa Huang is an associate professor at the Department of Internal Medicine, School of Medicine, Saint Louis University, Saint Louis, USA. After obtaining his PhD from Xiamen University, China, he joined the University of Texas Southwestern Medical Center, Dallas, Texas, as a postdoctoral fellow. In 2000, the American Heart Association awarded Dr. Huang a Scientist Development Grant. Over the decades, Dr. Huang's research focused on defining novel signaling pathways that regulate lipid metabolism and analyzing how lipid metabolism alters in the chemoimmunotherapeutic treatment. Dr. Huang's research has been supported by the American Veteran Affairs, the American Heart Association, and the National Institutes of Health. He has published over 50 peer-reviewed articles in scientific journals and several book chapters. He also served as an editorial board member and reviewer for a number of journals.

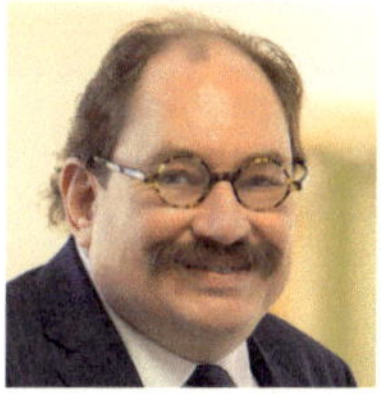

Dr. Carl Freter is a professor of Internal Medicine; division director, Hematology and Medical Oncology; and intern director, Cancer Center, Saint Louis University School of Medicine and also is a Rosalie Fusz Endowed Chair of Hematology at the Saint Louis University, Saint Louis, Missouri, USA. He received his MD and PhD from Washington University in Saint Louis. Dr. Freter was a resident at the Department of Internal Medicine, Stanford University Medical Center, and a fellow at the National Cancer Institute, National Institutes of Health. He was an assistant professor and associate professor at the Division of Medical Oncology, Department of Medicine, Georgetown University Medical Center, and a professor at the Ellis Fischel Cancer Center, University of Missouri, Columbia, Missouri. Dr. Freter's major interest is in cancer therapy and lipid metabolism, and he has conducted many basic and clinical research projects funded by the National Institutes of Health, various foundations, and drug companies. Dr. Freter has published numerous scientific papers in international journals and has written several chapters for different books on cancer.

Contents

Preface

Cholesterol is an essential component of cellular membranes and is involved in vesicle trafficking, receptor-mediated signaling, and steroidogenesis, which further lead to specific biological responses and regulate different cellular functions such as cell growth, proliferation, apoptosis, and migration as well as tumor progression. Alteration of cholesterol levels leads to pathophysiological changes. Hypercholesterolemia is a major risk factor for heart disease and stroke. Lowering cholesterol levels is an ideal strategy for preventing and reducing the burden of cardiovascular diseases. The development of cholesterol-lowering drugs is based on the modulation of cholesterol metabolism (synthesis and degradation), transportation (influx and efflux), and absorption and depletion. This book has the simple and singular mission of focusing on cholesterol-lowering drugs and their role in therapeutics. The book introduces different natural cholesterol busters and evaluates their actions. The book explores the development of pharmaceutical cholesterol-lowering drugs and their effects on the prevention and treatment of different diseases. The book also reviews the current knowledge in ethnic differences in response to cholesterol-lowering drug treatment. We have strived to present the readers current information on cholesterol-lowering drug development, evaluation, and therapeutic application.

These chapters have been written by prominent investigators in the field, and we thank the contributors for sharing their results and thoughts.

Dr. Chunfa Huang and Dr. Carl Freter
Division of Hematology and Medical Oncology,
Department of Internal Medicine, School of Medicine,
Saint Louis University, Saint Louis,
USA

Chapter 1

Natural Cholesterol Busters

Gamaleldin I. Harisa, Sabry M. Attia and
Gamil M. Abd Allah

Additional information is available at the end of the chapter

http://dx.doi.org/10.5772/64077

Abstract

Hypercholesterolemia, a risk factor for cardiovascular and cerebrovascular diseases, is a silent health problem. It occurs due to buildup of large amount of cholesterol in blood vessels resulting in narrowed blood vessels or blockage of the flow of blood and causes cellular dysfunction. The predisposing factors for hypercholesterolemia are carbohydrates-enriched diet, unhealthy fats, and red meat. Moreover, family history, obesity, hypokinetic lifestyle, aging, and oxidative stress are associated with hypercholesterolemia. Therapeutic interventions of hypercholesterolemia involve cessation of bad habits, regular exercise, consumption of cholesterol buster diets, and cholesterol-lowering drugs. However, cholesterol-lowering drugs have low efficacy, and some patients cannot tolerate the adverse effects of hypocholesterolemic drugs. In light of this, there has been great interest to address natural cholesterol busters as first choice as cholesterol-lowering option. Healthy diet, regular exercise and natural cholesterol-lowering agents are documented to decrease blood cholesterol level. Natural cholesterol busters include dietary fibers, plant sterols, healthy fats, smart proteins, antinutrients, antioxidants, and L-arginine. These busters not only decrease cholesterol oxidation and absorption but also increase cholesterol catabolism and elimination. Most of these busters are found in cereals, oatmeal, fruits, vegetables, legumes, and fermented foods. The natural cholesterol busters are recommended strategies for treatment of hypercholesterolemia alone or in combination with cholesterol-lowering drugs.

Keywords: hypercholesterolemia, health diet, antioxidants, antinutrients, cardiovascular diseases, L-arginine

1. Introduction

Cholesterol is an important component in cell membrane that maintains the structure and function of the cells. Moreover, cholesterol is a precursor of sex hormones, corticosteroid, and vitamin D. This vitamin is involved in bone formation, modulates immune system, and regulates gene expression [1]. Cholesterol can be catabolized into bile acids that play an important role in digestion and absorption of fat diets and fat-soluble vitamins. The cells get its cholesterol through two pathways, endogenous source by means of biosynthesis in liver (80 %) and exogenous source from the diet (20%) [2]. Cholesterol is transported throughout the bloodstream by joining to specific proteins and lipids forming lipoproteins. There are four main types of lipoprotein acting as cholesterol carriers in circulation: chylomicrons, very low-density lipoproteins (VLDL), low-density lipoprotein (LDL) "bad cholesterol", and high-density lipoprotein (HDL) "good cholesterol" [1].

HDL elicits cardioprotective function by reverse cholesterol transport to the liver to be catabolized, moreover, HDL has antioxidant and anti-inflammatory effects as well as involved in nitric oxide (NO) homeostasis [3]. Under hypercholesterolemic conditions, HDL can be turned into a foe for vascular endothelium through production of free radicals that induced vascular cells and erythrocytes damage [3]. Moreover, cholesterol enrichment decreases membrane fluidity, disrupts cell signaling, induces toxic oxysterols, modulates gene expression, and induces apoptosis [4]. This results in disruption of redox balance and NO homeostasis, particularly in vascular cells and erythrocytes. Cholesterol-enriched erythrocyte membrane causes a reduction in the deformability of cells and impairment of the hemorheological behavior that can initiate cardiovascular disease [5]. Oxidative stress is one of the proposed mechanisms responsible for the changes in erythrocytes under hypercholesterolemic conditions; hence, erythrocytes lose their antioxidant power and become oxidized erythrocytes, which triggers foam cell formation by a mechanism similar to oxidized lipoproteins [5]. Therefore, oxidized erythrocytes are addressed as a new culprit in vascular diseases. **Figure 1** displays the double face of cholesterol.

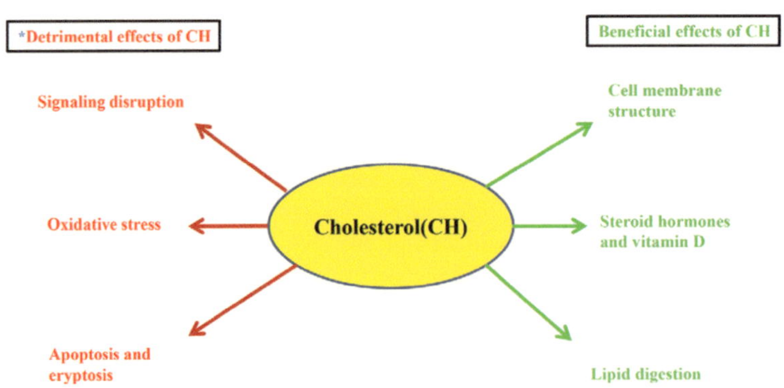

Figure 1. Beneficial and detrimental effects of cholesterol. Asterisk indicates hypercholesterolemic conditions.

http://dx.doi.org/10.5772/64077

Cholesterol-lowering drug therapies particularly with cholesterol biosynthesis inhibitors are associated with adverse effects such as myopathies, neuropathies, liver dysfunction, weakness, and depression [6]. However, intake of natural cholesterol busters reduces blood cholesterol level with minimal side effects [7–9]. Natural cholesterol busters include healthy diet—drinking excess cold water and avoidance of stress with regular exercise. Moreover, many nutraceuticals have cholesterol-lowering action; they include dietary fibers, plant sterols, healthy fats, smart proteins, antinutrients, antioxidants, and L-arginine [10]. These busters act by modulation biochemical pathways such as appetite suppression, inhibition of digestion, and absorption of dietary fats. In addition, they not only increase the metabolic rate and lipolysis but also decrease lipogenesis and inhibit adipocyte differentiation. **Figure 2** shows the possible mechanisms by which natural cholesterol-lowering agents decrease plasma cholesterol levels.

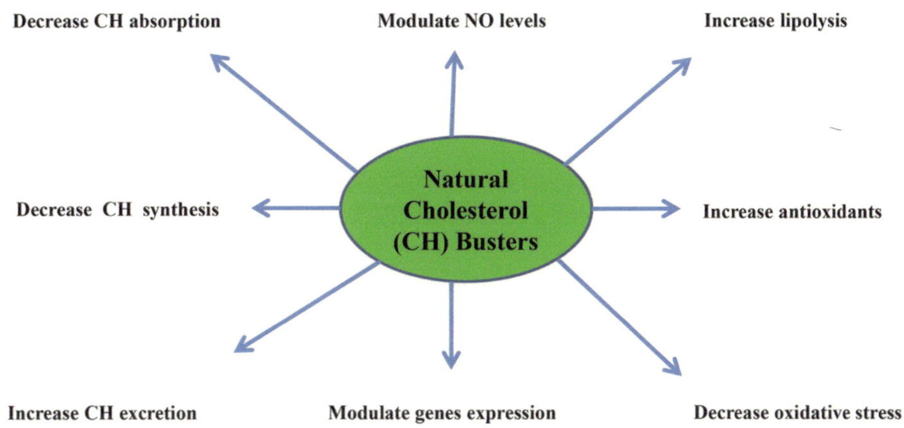

Figure 2. Beneficial effects of natural cholesterol busters.

On this basis, the selection of natural cholesterol-lowering agents with dual action such as lipid lowering and antioxidant activities with minimal side effects is very essential. Natural cholesterol busters can reduce blood cholesterol levels and risk of vascular diseases without adverse effects. This chapter highlights natural cholesterol busters as first line of cholesterol-lowering strategy.

2. Natural cholesterol busters

The first choice to decrease the blood cholesterol levels is lifestyle change including healthy diet—drinking excess of water, avoidance of stress and regular exercise. Moreover, there are a group of nutraceuticals that can be considered as cholesterol busters. Some of these nutraceuticals are plant sterols, healthy fats, dietary fibers, antinutrients, antioxidants, and L-arginine.

2.1. Healthy lifestyle as natural cholesterol busters

2.1.1. Health diet and exercise

Diet and lifestyle are major causes of dyslipidemia, diabetes, and cardiovascular diseases. Particularly, protein-enriched diet produces satiating effect and helps stave off hunger [10]. Consumption of plant-based foods lowers the rate of many chronic diseases; this is attributable to diets which contain smart proteins, trace elements, foliate, antioxidants, and antinutrients [10]. Additionally, low carbohydrate consumption modulates hormones release, increases lipolysis, and enhances fatty acids oxidation [10]. On the other hand, aerobic exercise decreases lipogenesis and activates lipoprotein lipase that increases lipolysis, resulted in enhancement of fat clearance and burning [11].

In these situations, depot fats and free fatty acids were utilized as fuel sources for muscle work [12]. Therefore, health diet with regular exercise (3h/week) at least for 5 days per week decreases subcutaneous fats, visceral fats as well as improve blood lipid levels [12]. Generally, the reduction of body fats is associated with a decrease of total cholesterol, triacylglycerol, LDL, while HDL levels were increased [10]. Furthermore, health diet and lifestyle modifications improve the availability of nitric oxide [10]. Therefore, healthy diets enriched with plant protein, low in carbohydrate and fat, devoid of trans fats (margarine, snack food, packaged baked food, and fried fast food), with regular exercise could be considered the best choice to treat hypercholesterolemia. Besides the aforementioned effects, caloric restrictions with exercise preserve antioxidant capacity as well as reduce reactive oxygen species formation and reduce apoptosis.

2.1.2. Cessation of bad habits

Cigarette smoking and alcohol drinking are most common bad habits worldwide. Combined use of both smoking and alcohol is more damaging to health than use of either alone. The most serious medical consequences of smoking and alcohol are vascular diseases and cancer [13]. This attribute of cigarette smoking enhances catecholamine release and inhibits lipoprotein lipase activity; this results in an increase in levels of chylomicrons, VLDL, and LDL with a decrease in HDL levels [14]. These resulted in alteration of lipid profile associated with decline of antioxidant power with an increase of lipid peroxidation, thrombosis, and vascular dysfunction [13]. Smoking cessation averts these deleterious effects on lipid abnormality, particularly HDL levels [14].

The liver plays a central role in the regulation of cholesterol homeostasis. Alcohol drinking causes fatty liver, besides this alcohol is metabolized into acetaldehyde and reactive oxygen radicals [15]. Acetaldehyde and reactive oxygen radicals can interact with proteins, lipids, and other biomolecules in the cell, resulting in adduct formation which is harmful to the liver. Moreover, acetaldehyde-protein adducts upregulate lipogenetic genes in the liver [15]. Several studies confirmed that chronic alcoholism induced abnormality in lipid metabolism with elevation of triacylglycerol and cholesterol-enriched lipoproteins in the blood [16].

2.2. Nutraceutical as natural cholesterol busters

2.2.1. Healthy fats

Dietary fatty acids are considered one of the main important dietary supplements that strongly determine the development of cardiovascular diseases. The dietary fatty acids include saturated fatty acids, monounsaturated fatty acids, and polyunsaturated fatty acids (PUFAs) [17]. Saturated fatty acid–rich diets are implicated in the promotion of cardiovascular diseases, while monounsaturated fatty acids and PUFAs have cardioprotective effects [17]. In particular, PUFAs are essential dietary elements for human body because human body lacks desaturating enzymes that are required for PUFAs' biosynthesis [18].

PUFAs are classified according to the position of first double bond from the methyl end (omega carbon) into omega-3 ($\omega 3$) PUFAs and omega-6 ($\omega 6$) PUFAs. Dietary intake of $\omega 3$-PUFAs with reduction in $\omega 6$-PUFAs consumption is beneficial for cardiac health [19], while higher consumption of $\omega 6$-PUFAs with lower $\omega 3$-PUFAs dietary contents is a risk for many diseases, particularly cardiovascular diseases. Inside the human body α-linolenic acid can be converted to eicosapentaenoic acid and docosahexaenoic acid by desaturase and elongase enzymes in a series of biochemical reactions [20]. The process of endogenous desaturation and elongation of α-linolenic acid into eicosapentaenoic acid and docosahexaenoic acid is usually inefficient. Therefore, intake of α-linolenic acid is essential for production of eicosapentaenoic and docosahexaenoic acids [21–24].

Omega-3 fatty acids are the precursors of biologically active mediators with health benefits with regard to their anti-inflammatory, antithrombotic, hypolipidemic, and cardioprotective effects [20]. However, $\omega 6$-PUFA produces pro-inflammatory, pro-thrombotic, and pro-atherogenic mediators [21–24]. Therefore, balanced ratio between $\omega 3$-PUFAs/$\omega 6$-PUFAs dietary intake is recommended for the decrease of cardiovascular risk. The reversal of this ratio has been considered responsible for the high prevalence of cardiovascular disease [21–24].

The $\omega 3$-PUFAs are involved in the formation of phospholipids that are involved in reverse cholesterol transport to the liver for catabolism [24]. Additionally, intake of $\omega 3$-PUFAs can reduce triacylglycerol levels through inhibition of hepatic lipogenesis and very low-density lipoproteins production by the liver and output into circulation. The $\omega 3$-PUFAs have been shown to increase plasma LDL with large particle size, which is much less atherogenic than LDL that cannot infiltrate blood vessels of vascular endothelium to start development of atherosclerosis [24]. Moreover, $\omega 3$-PUFAs downregulate sterol regulatory element-binding protein, resulting in suppression of gene expression of 3-hydroxy-3-methyl-glutaryl CoA reductase, a rate-limiting enzyme in cholesterol synthesis [25]. $\omega 3$-PUFAs also activate liver X receptors that upregulate expression of 7-α-hydroxylase, the main enzyme in conversion of cholesterol into bile acids [26].

Diet enriched with $\omega 3$-PUFAs is abundant in plant and marine sources, such as flaxseed, canola, salmon, mackerel, herring, and tuna. The fish oil is composed of higher percent of $\omega 3$-PUFAs; therefore, they are the best source of biologically active $\omega 3$-PUFAs mediators. The $\omega 3$-PUFAs have susceptibility to oxidative damage; therefore, antioxidants supplementation is recommended during ω3-PUFAs consumption. The ω3-PUFAs are promising therapeutic options for the prevention and treatment of hypercholesterolemia. The risk of antioxidants deficiency and mercury contamination during intake of fish oils must be considered.

2.2.2. *Phytosterols*

Phytosterols are plant source sterols; they are similar to animal sterol in the presence of steroid nucleus, whereas they differ in their side chain. Phytosterols have been incorporated in many dietary regimens to reduce plasma cholesterol levels and provide a cardioprotective action [27–28]. Phytosterols are classified according to their saturation into sterols and stanols; saturation of sterols produces stanols. The main physterols are sitosterol and campesterol, with their respective stanols, sitostanol and campestanol [27–28]. Phytosterols are relatively less absorbed than cholesterol, particularly stanols. Addition of phytosterols to the diet of hypercholesterolemic patients can effectively reduce blood cholesterol levels [29–30]. Phytostanols are preferred than sterols because the effect of sterols diminishes over time, while stanols' effect persists for a long time. Maximal reduction in cholesterol was reported with daily intake of 2.0 g of plant stanols. The effect of phytosterols is food dependent because the maximal bile secretion is with or directly after meals where stanols can target micelle formation to reduce the absorption of cholesterol and lipids [31–35]. Phytostanols esters showed greater effectiveness if taken on daily basis in sufficient amounts (0.8–2.0 g) with meals [31–35]. The beneficial effect of stanols over LDL reduction appears after 1–2 weeks of (2.0 g) daily consumption. Most importantly, this reduction in LDL persists as long as stanols being consumed [31–35].

Several mechanisms including interference with intestinal cholesterol solubility, inhibition of digestive enzymes, and decreasing cellular uptake of cholesterol have been proposed to explain the cholesterol-lowering effects of phytosterols [31–35]. Therefore, phytosterols reduce the absorption of both dietary and biliary cholesterol from the intestinal tract. Moreover, phytosterols induce the expression of ATP-binding cassette transporters, thus increasing the efflux of cholesterol from the intestinal cells [31–35]. In addition, phytosterols suppress the activity of acyl-cholesterol acyl transferase required for sterols absorption, consequently reducing intestinal cholesterol uptake. Phytosterols are partially inhibiting dietary and biliary cholesterol absorption by 30–50% through inhibition of cholesterol emulsification through disruption of the lipid micelles, reducing its solubility and availability for intestinal absorption [31–35]. Phytosterols are present naturally in many plants, such as corn, soybeans, and sunflower seeds. The risk of beta-sitosterolemia must be considered during intake of phytosterols as cholesterol-lowering therapy.

2.2.3. *Dietary fibers*

Dietary fibers including cellulose and its derivatives as well as lignin are considered as non-digestible parts of food. Diet rich in fiber has been reported to have an inverse relationship to cardiovascular risk. Therefore, fiber-enriched diets are recommended by many leading organizations to improve human health [36–37]. The chemical composition of dietary fibers is carbohydrate in nature; they are present in edible plants. Dietary fibers resist alimentary digestive enzymes, are non-absorbable and susceptible for partial fermentation by normal flora gastrointestinal tract [36–37]. Generally, dietary fibers are classified according to their solubility into soluble and insoluble fibers. Inulin, oligofructosides, pectin, mucilage, psyllium, gum, polysaccharides, and β-glucans are examples for soluble fibers, whereas lignin, cellulose, hemicellulose, and resistant starch are examples for insoluble fibers [38–41]. Chitosan can reduce the risk of cardiovascular diseases because it can lower triacylglycerol and cholesterol levels by increasing bile acid excretion [42].

Dietary fibers have hypolipidemic effect over both triacylglycerol and cholesterol-enriched lipoproteins [41]. The biochemical mechanisms underlying the hypolipidemic effect of dietary fibers may be due to different hypotheses. Dietary fibers form complexes with dietary fats, cholesterol, and bile acids. Therefore, fat digestion by pancreatic lipases is inhibited, while hepatic bile synthesis and cholesterol excretion are enhanced [41, 43]. In addition, dietary fibers can entrap water and water-soluble foodstuff, such as glucose, resulting in reduction in glucose absorption. Therefore, post-prandial plasma insulin declines with suppression of its stimulating action for 3-hydroxy-3-methylglutaryl-CoA reductase in cholesterol synthesis. This resulted in decrease of cholesterol biosynthesis with decrease in blood cholesterol levels [41, 43]. Fermentation of fibers by intestinal flora produces short chain fatty acids such as propionic and butyric acids. These acids can suppress hepatic cholesterol synthesis via competitive inhibition of 3-hydroxy-3-methyl-glutaryl CoA reductase and downregulate most of lipogenic enzymes [41, 43–45].

Dietary fibers promote growth of intestinal microflora such as *Lactobacillus acidophilus* [37]. Therefore, dietary fibers that selectively stimulate the growth and activity of beneficial microflora are known as "prebiotics"; "probiotics" in the gastrointestinal tract improve the intestinal microbial balance, thus improving human health. When probiotics and prebiotics are used in combination, they are known as "synbiotics" [46]. The use of synbiotics is to improve gut health and exert other health-promoting effects, such as modulation of the immune system, antihypertensive effects, prevention of cancer, antioxidant effects, reduction of dermatitis symptoms, facilitation of mineral absorption, and improvement of candidiasis [46]. Additionally, synbiotics has cholesterol-lowering properties through deconjugation of bile acids by bile-salt hydrolase, thus leading to coprecipitation of cholesterol with deconjugated bile [46]. Other explanations for cholesterol-lowering effects of probiotics include utilization of cholesterol in the cell membranes during growth of probiotics, conversion of cholesterol into coprostanol and production of short-chain fatty acids upon prebiotics fermentation by probiotics [46].

Dietary fibers are present in nuts, beans, lentil, lupin, blueberries, cucumber, green leafy vegetables, green beans, carrot, celery, yoghurt, and fermented foods.

2.2.4. *Antioxidants*

Antioxidants can minimize cellular damage by inactivating free radicals, which could attack other cellular molecules. Enzymatic antioxidants that could provide a protection against free radicals are superoxide dismutase, catalase, and glutathione peroxidases [47]. Non-enzymatic antioxidants with similar function are present widely in the biological system and able to quench many types of free radicals. They include glutathione, vitamin E, vitamin C, β-carotene, retinols, selenium, copper, zinc, manganese, and others [47]. Hypercholesterolemia upregulates the activity of free radical–generating enzymes; however, it downregulates the activity of antioxidant enzymes that trigger the production of reactive oxygen metabolites [48]. These reactive metabolites provoke lipoproteins oxidation, protein glycation, and glucose autooxidation. Therefore, hypercholesterolemia has been implicated as pathogenesis of pancreatitis, hepatitis, renal injury, stroke, atherosclerosis, and metabolic syndrome by oxidative damage-dependent mechanism [49].

There are scientific evidences of the protective effects of naturally occurring antioxidants in biological systems. Consequently, the identification of natural antioxidants with cholesterol-lowering effect in diet consumed by human is very important. Antioxidants are attractive alternative therapy to treat hypercholesterolemic patients [50]. The antioxidants with cholesterol-lowering capability include antioxidant vitamins, coenzymeQ-10, resveratrol, grape seed, cherry seed, and spices. Moreover, flavonoids, such as silymarin, rutin, quercetin, naringin, and hesperidin, were used for the same purpose [7–9]. Chrysin is a natural flavonoid that is able to decrease plasma lipid concentration and has an antioxidant property [51]. Moreover, rice bran oil is involved in lipid metabolism and oxidation; therefore, it has significant health benefits by the modulation of lipid profiles and preservation of normal redox balance in hypercholesterolemic conditions [52]. Antioxidants are exerting their beneficial effects as free radical scavengers and as chelators of pro-oxidant metals. Furthermore, administration of antioxidants augments endogenous antioxidant power as well as inhibits free radicals generating enzymes [54]. Antioxidants inhibit the oxidation of lipoproteins, protect the oxidative damage of erythrocytes and preserve the availability of nitric oxide in the body [53]. Consequently, antioxidants prevent hypercholesterolemia-induced vascular cells damage. Vegetables and fruits are good source of antioxidants; they include reddish, lettuce, carrot, tomato, cucumber, red cabbage, and low caloric fruits such as apple, grape fruits and orange.

2.2.5. Antinutrients

Antinutrients are plant secondary metabolites such as saponins, flavonoids, alkaloids, tannins, oxalates, phytates, protease inhibitors, amylase inhibitors, lipase inhibitors, and lectins. They are secreted by the plant as a part of the defense mechanism [54, 55]. Human beings use these agents for many beneficial purposes. Some of the antinutrients are used in modulation of gastrointestinal function. Lectins have high binding capacity to the intestinal brush border membrane. This stimulates the release of anorectic neuropeptides that produce satiety and decrease food intake [55]. However, lectins can cause severe intestinal damage with disrupting digestion provoking food allergies and other immune responses [55]. Saponins are amphipathic antinutrients which can reduce cholesterol absorption by disruption of cholesterol micelle formation and downregulate the activity of lipogenic enzymes [54, 55]. Furthermore, saponins also reduce the uptake of glucose from the gut through intraluminal physicochemical interaction [54, 55].

Tannins are present in most cereals and are able to inhibit the activities of protease, amylase and lipase [54–56]. Chlorogenic acid is a member of antinutrients present in green coffee.

Soybeans, fenugreek, bean, and ginseng are good sources of antinutrients. Antinutrients have immune-potentiating action, anticancer effect, and antioxidant power, which could prevent cardiovascular diseases. However, the risk of hemolysis, pancreatic hypertrophy, minerals deficiency, vitamins deficiency, and other malabsorption syndrome must be considered during intake of antinutrients for treatment of hypercholesterolemia [54–56]. **Table 1** annotated the common dietary sources, the main mechanisms of action, and the probable side effects of natural cholesterol lowering agents.

Cholesterol buster	Dietary source	Main mechanism of action	Probable side effects
Healthy fats	Salmon, flaxseed, and canola oils	Decrease cholesterol synthesis and increase its catabolism	Depletion of antioxidant
Phytosterols	Corn, soybeans, and sunflower seeds	Induce expression of ATP-binding cassette transporters	Beta-Sitosterolemia
Dietary fibers	Legumes, beans, and vegetables	Form complexes with dietary cholesterol and bile acids	Abdominal discomfort
Antinutrients	Beans, fenugreek, and ginseng	Produce satiety and decrease cholesterol micelles formation	Hemolysis and malabsorption syndrome
Antioxidants	Fruits, vegetables, and rice bran oil	Decrease free radicals formation and lipoprotein oxidation	-
L-arginine	Poultry, seafood, and lupine	Antioxidants and restores nitric oxide bioavailability	Hypotension

Table 1. The common dietary sources, the main mechanisms of action, and the probable side effects of natural cholesterol busters.

2.2.6. L-Arginine

Nitric oxide is an important vasodilator and has many biological functions. Several cells including endothelial cells and erythrocytes can produce nitric oxide which uses L-arginine as a substrate and tetrahydrobiopterin and flavoproteins as cofactors [57, 58]. Hypercholesterolemia is associated with the increased oxidative stress that reduces the nitric oxide bioavailability through disruption of L-arginine transport into cells, inactivation of nitric oxide synthase, and activation of arginase [9, 58, 59]. Furthermore, high blood cholesterol levels increase endogenous L-arginine analogues that are able to inhibit nitric oxide synthesis. In particular, asymmetric dimethylarginine competes with L-arginine at the catalytic site of nitric oxide synthase, and symmetric dimethylarginine blocks the transport of L-arginine into the cells via the transporter for cationic amino acids [9, 58, 59]. In hypercholesterolemia, erythrocytes and endothelial cells float in cholesterol-enriched media. This results in a decrease of nitric oxide production and endothelial dysfunction [9, 58, 59]. On the contrary, L-arginine supplementation restores nitric oxide levels and reduces vascular oxidative damage in hypercholesterolemic conditions [57]. It has been reported that L-arginine–enriched foods lower LDL levels; this indicates positive health benefits associated with L-arginine on cardiovascular system [60]. Moreover, dietary supplementation with L-arginine stimulates nitric oxide biosynthetic pathway. In addition, polyphenolic compound mediates L-arginine transport into cells and enhances nitric oxide production [60, 61]. L-arginine–enriched foods include dairy products, poultry, seafood, wheat germ, lupine, granola, oatmeal, peanuts, nuts, pumpkin seed, and chickpeas. The risk of hypotension must be considered during intake of L-arginine as a cholesterol-lowering agent. **Figure 3** shows role of cholesterol busters in prevention hypercholesterolemia induced endothelial dysfunction.

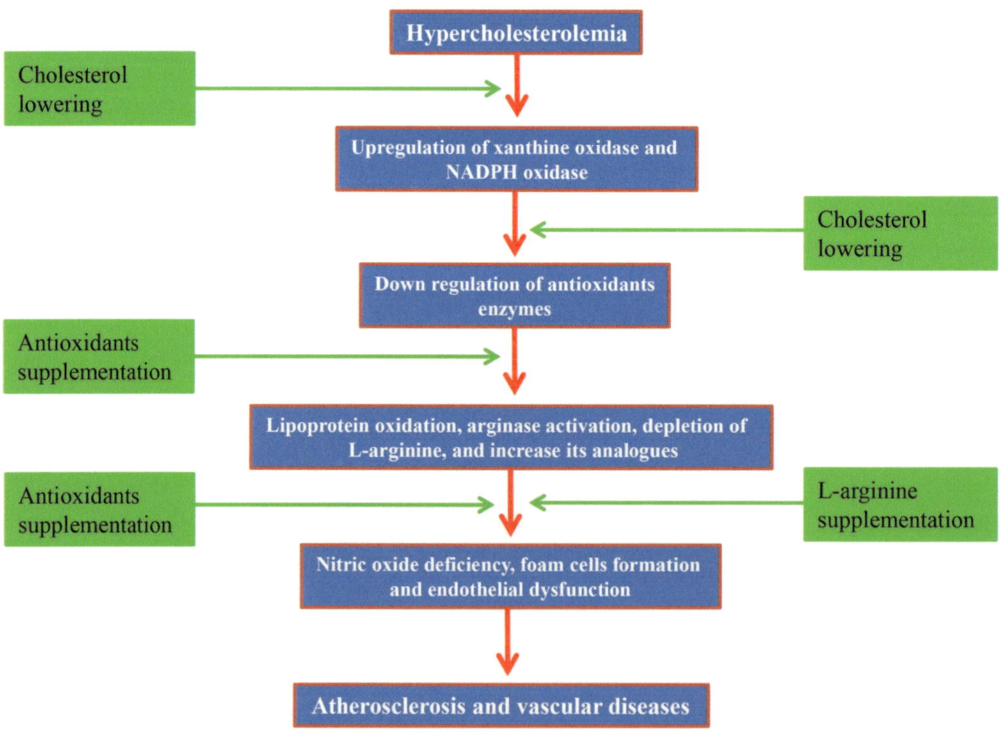

Figure 3. Mechanisms of action of cholesterol busters in prevention hypercholesterolemia induced endothelial dysfunction. Green color indicates the site of action of therapeutic agent.

3. Suggestion and recommendations

Based on the current data in this chapter, the following recommendations aid in maintaining a healthy life.

- Eat three to five healthy diet daily containing different foods. Healthy diets contain fruits, vegetables, and legumes with less fat and carbohydrate.
- Reduce the intake of salt, flour, and sugar; use more fibers and reduce the amount of food in your plate.
- Consume cold water and sugar-free gum during a feeling of false or emotional hunger.
- Motivate regularly such as walking, riding a bike, and other activities (30–45 min), at least 5 days weekly to burn off the excess calories.
- Prohibit bad habits such smoking and alcohol drinking as conceivable.
- Avoid overcrowding, noise, and contaminant exposure as possible.
- Check your body weight weekly.
- Examine your blood sugar level and plasma lipids profile for every 6 months.

4. Summary

Healthy diet and exercise can successfully manage blood cholesterol levels, besides supplementation of natural cholesterol busters. Natural cholesterol busters not only decrease cholesterol absorption, but also increase cholesterol metabolism and elimination. The intervention of natural cholesterol busters is the safest strategy in the prevention and treatment of hypercholesterolemia. The hypocholesterolemic properties of natural cholesterol busters have been proved; however, further studies are required to address general recommendations considering human variability in response to dietary regimen. The natural cholesterol busters are found in cereals, oatmeal, fruits, vegetables, and legumes. In case of failure of natural cholesterol busters as first choice cholesterol-lowering option, the cholesterol-lowering drugs are recommended with natural cholesterol busters. Take care that high intake of antinutrients may be associated with serious health problems due to the presence of phytate, oxalate, cyanogenic glycoside, and other toxic antinutrients.

Acknowledgements

The authors extend their appreciation to Kayyali Chair for Pharmaceutical Industry, Department of Pharmaceutics, College of Pharmacy, King Saud University for funding this work through the research project Number (G-2016-1).

Author details

Gamaleldin I. Harisa[1,3*], Sabry M. Attia[2] and Gamil M. Abd Allah[3]

*Address all correspondence to: harisa@ksu.edu.sa

1 Kayyali Chair for Pharmaceutical Industry, College of Pharmacy, King Saud University, Riyadh, Saudi Arabia

2 Department of Pharmacology and Toxicology, College of Pharmacy, King Saud University, Riyadh, Saudi Arabia

3 Department of Biochemistry, College of Pharmacy, Al-Azhar University (Boys), Nasr City, Cairo, Egypt

References

[1] Widmaier E, Raff H, Strang K. Vander's human physiology: the mechanisms of body function. 13th ed. New York, NY: McGraw-Hill Science/Engineering/Math; 2013.

[2] Ikonen E. Cellular cholesterol trafficking and compartmentalization. Nat Rev Mol Cell Biol. 2008; 9(2):125–38.

[3] Xu S, Liu Z, Liu P. HDL cholesterol in cardiovascular diseases: the good, the bad, and the ugly? Int J Cardiol. 2013; 168(4):3157–9.

[4] Tabas I. Consequences of cellular cholesterol accumulation: basic concepts and physiological implications. J Clin Invest. 2002; 110(7):905–11.

[5] Harisa GI, Badran M, Alanazi F, Attia S, Shazly G. Influence of pravastatin chitosan nanoparticles on erythrocytes cholesterol and redox homeostasis: an in vitro study. Arab J Chem. 2015; http://dx.doi.org/10.1016/j.arabjc.2015.10.016. In press.

[6] Petyaev IM. Improvement of hepatic bioavailability as a new step for the future of statin. Arch Med Sci. 2015; 11(2):406–10.

[7] Franiak-Pietryga I, Koter-Michalak M, Broncel M, Duchnowicz P, Chojnowska-Jezierska J. Anti-inflammatory and hypolipemic effects in vitro of simvastatin comparing to epicatechin in patients with type-2 hypercholesterolemia. Food Chem Toxicol. 2009; 47(2):393–7.

[8] Duchnowicz P, Bors M, Podsędek A, Koter-Michalak M, Broncel M. Effect of polyphenols extracts from Brassica vegetables on erythrocyte membranes (in vitro study). Environ Toxicol Pharmacol. 2012; 34(3):783–90.

[9] Csonka C, Sárközy M, Pipicz M, Dux L, Csont T. Modulation of hypercholesterolemia-induced oxidative/nitrative stress in the heart. Oxid Med Cell Longev. 2016;3863726.

[10] Harisa GI, Alanazi FK. The beneficial roles of Lupineus luteus and lifestyle changes in management of metabolic syndrome: a case study. Saudi Pharm J. 2015; 23(6):712–5.

[11] Plaisance EP, Fisher G. Exercise and dietary-mediated reductions in postprandial lipemia. J Nutr Metab. 2014;902065.

[12] Togashi K, Masuda H, Iguchi K. Effect of diet and exercise treatment for obese Japanese children on abdominal fat distribution. Res Sports Med. 2010; 18(1):62–70.

[13] McCullough ML, Patel AV, Kushi LH, Patel R, Willett WC, Doyle C, Thun MJ, Gapstur SM. Following cancer prevention guidelines reduces risk of cancer, cardiovascular disease, and all-cause mortality. Cancer Epidemiol. Biomarkers Prev. 2011; 20(6):1089–97.

[14] Chelland Campbell S, Moffatt RJ, Stamford BA. Smoking and smoking cessation the relationship between cardiovascular disease and lipoprotein metabolism: a review. Atherosclerosis. 2008; 201(2):225–35.

[15] Oliva J, French SW, Li J, Bardag-Gorce F. Proteasome inhibitor treatment reduced fatty acid, triacylglycerol and cholesterol synthesis. Exp Mol Pathol. 2012; 93(1):26–34.

[16] Wang Z, Yao T, Song Z. Chronic alcohol consumption disrupted cholesterol homeostasis in rats: down-regulation of low-density lipoprotein receptor and enhancement of cholesterol biosynthesis pathway in the liver. Alcohol Clin Exp Res. 2010; 34(3):471–8.

[17] Gillingham LG, Harris-Janz S, Jones PJ. Dietary monounsaturated fatty acids are protective against metabolic syndrome and cardiovascular disease risk factors. Lipids. 2011; 46:209–28.

[18] Engler MM, Engler MB. Omega-3 fatty acids: role in cardiovascular health and disease. J Cardiovasc Nurs. 2006; 21:17–24; quiz 25–6.

[19] Grenon SM, Hughes-Fulford M, Rapp J, Conte MS. Polyunsaturated fatty acids and peripheral artery disease. Vasc Med. 2012; 17:51–63.

[20] Seo T, Blaner WS, Deckelbaum RJ. Omega-3 fatty acids: molecular approaches to optimal biological outcomes. Curr Opin Lipidol. 2005; 16:11–8.

[21] Brenna JT. Efficiency of conversion of alpha-linolenic acid to long chain *n*–3 fatty acids in man. Curr Opin Clin Nutr Metab Care. 2002; 5:127–32.

[22] Adkins Y, Kelley DS. Mechanisms underlying the cardioprotective effects of omega-3 polyunsaturated fatty acids. J NutrBiochem. 2010; 21:781–92.

[23] Gomez Candela C, Bermejo Lopez LM, Loria Kohen V. Importance of a balanced omega 6/omega 3 ratio for the maintenance of health: nutritional recommendations. Nutr Hosp. 2011; 26:323–9.

[24] Balogun K, & Cheema S. Cardioprotective role of omega-3 polyunsaturated fatty acids through the regulation of lipid metabolism. Ch. 27 in: Jagadeesh J, et al. (editors). Pathophysiology and pharmacotherapy cardiovascular disease. 1st ed. 2015. Aids (an imprint of Springer), Germany.

[25] Le Jossic-Corcos C, Gonthier C, Zaghini I, Logette E, Shechter I, Bournot P. Hepatic farnesyl diphosphate synthase expression is suppressed by polyunsaturated fatty acids. Biochem J. 2005; 385:787–94.

[26] Davidson MH. Mechanisms for the hypotriglyceridemic effect of marine omega-3 fatty acids. Am J Cardiol. 2006; 98:27i–33.

[27] Genser B, Silbernagel G, De Backer G, Bruckert E, Carmena R, Chapman MJ et al. Plant sterols and cardiovascular disease: a systematic review and meta-analysis. Eur Heart J. 2012; 33(4):444–51.

[28] Thompson GR, Grundy SM. History and development of plant sterol and stanol esters for cholesterol-lowering purposes. Am J Cardiol. 2005; 96(Suppl):3D–9D.

[29] O'Neill FH, Sanders TA, Thompson GR. Comparison of efficacy of plant stanol ester and sterol ester: short-term and longer-term studies. Am J Cardiol. 2005; 96(1A):29D–36D.

[30] Miettinen TA, Gylling H. Effect of statins on noncholesterol sterol levels: implications for use of plant stanols and sterols. Am J Cardiol. 2005; 96(1A):40D–6D.

[31] Cater NB, Garcia-Garcia AB, Vega GL, Grundy SM. Responsiveness of plasma lipids and lipoproteins to plant stanol esters. Am J Cardiol 2005; 96(Suppl): 23D–8D.

[32] Assmann G, Seedorf U. Phytosterols, plasma lipids and CVD risk. Ch. 29 in: Mancini M, et al. (editors). Nutritional and metabolic bases of cardiovascular disease. 1st ed. 2011. Blackwell Publishing Limited, USA.

[33] Rosin S, Ojansivu I, Kopu A, Keto-Tokoi M, Gylling H. Optimal use of plant stanol ester in the management of hypercholesterolemia. Cholesterol. 2015; 2015:706970.

[34] King ED. Dietary fiber, inflammation, and cardiovascular disease. Mol Nutr Food Res. 2005; 49(6):594–600.

[35] Mudagil D, Barak S. Composition, properties and health benefits of indigestible carbohydrate polymers as dietary fiber: a review. Int J Biol Macromol. 2013; 61:1–6.

[36] Papathanasopoulos A, Camilleri M. Dietary fiber supplements: effects in obesity and metabolic syndrome and relationship to gastrointestinal functions. Gastroenterology. 2010; 138:65–72.

[37] Slavin JL. Carbohydrates, dietary fiber, and resistant starch in white vegetables: links to health outcomes. Adv Nutr. 2013; 4:351S–15S.

[38] Cani PD, Possemiers S, Van de Wiele T, et al. Changes in gut microbiota control inflammation in obese mice through a mechanism involving GLP-2-driven improvement of gut permeability. Gut. 2009; 58(8):1091–103.

[39] Urías-Silvas JE, Cani PD, Delmée E, Neyrinck A, López MG, Delzenne NM. Physiological effects of dietary fructans extracted from Agave tequilanaGto and Dasylirion spp. Br J Nutr. 2008; 99(2):254–61.

[40] Retelny VS, Neuendorf A, Roth JL. Nutrition protocols for the prevention of cardiovascular disease. Nutr Clin Pract. 2008; 23(5):468–76.

[41] Theuwissen E, Mensink RP. Water-soluble dietary fibers and cardiovascular disease. Physiol Behav. 2008; 94(2):285–92.

[42] Xia, W. Liu P, Zhang J, Chen J. Biological activities of chitosan and chitooligosaccharides. Food Hydrocoll. 2011; 25:170–9.

[43] Giovane A, Napoli C. Protective effects of food on cardiovascular disease. Ch. 24 in: Sauer H, et al. (editors). Studies on cardiovascular disorders. 2010. Humana Press (an imprint of Springer), USA.

[44] Artiss JD, Brogan K, Brucal M, Moghaddam M, Jen KL. The effects of a new soluble dietary fiber on weight gain and selected blood parameters in rats. Metabolism. 2006; 55(2):195–202.

[45] Delzenne NM, Williams CM. Prebiotics and lipid metabolism. Curr Opin Lipidol. 2002; 13(1):61–67.

[46] Ooi LG, Liong MT. Cholesterol-lowering effects of probiotics and prebiotics: a review of in vivo and in vitro findings. Int J Mol Sci. 2010; 11(6):2499–522.

[47] Chitra KP, KS Pillai. Antioxidants in health. Ind J Physiol Pharmacol. 2002; 46(1):1–5.

[48] Costa LG1, Giordano G, Furlong CE. Pharmacological and dietary modulators of paraoxonase 1 (PON1) activity and expression: the hunt goes on. Biochem Pharmacol. 2011; 81(3):337–44.

[49] Olorunnisola OS, Bradley G, Afolayan AJ. Protective effect of T. violacea rhizome extract against hypercholesterolemia-induced oxidative stress in Wistar rats. Molecules. 2012; 17(5):6033–45.

[50] Deng R. Food and food supplements with hypocholesterolemic effects. Recent Pat Food Nutr Agric. 2009; 1(1):15–24.

[51] Zarzecki, MS, Araujo SM, Bortolotto VC, de Paula MT. Hypolipidemic action of chrysin on Triton WR-1339-induced hyperlipidemia in female C57BL/6 mice. Toxicol Rep. 2014; 1:200–8.

[52] Minhajuddin M1, Beg ZH, Iqbal J. Hypolipidemic and antioxidant properties of tocotrienol rich fraction isolated from rice bran oil in experimentally induced hyperlipidemic rats. Food Chem Toxicol. 2005; 43(5):747–53.

[53] Vogiatzi G, Tousoulis D, Stefanadis C. The role of oxidative stress in atherosclerosis. Hell J Cardiol. 2009; 50(5):402–9.

[54] Soetan KO. Pharmacological and other beneficial effects of antinutritional factors in plants: a review. Afr J Biotechnol 2008; 7(25):4713–21.

[55] Ramírez-Jiménez AK, Reynoso-Camacho R, Elizabeth Tejero M, León-Galván F, Loarca-Piña G. Potential role of bioactive compounds of *Phaseolus vulgaris L.* on lipid-lowering mechanisms. Food Res Int 2015; 7692–104.

[56] Meng S, Cao J, Feng Q, Peng J, Hu Y. Roles of chlorogenic acid on regulating glucose and lipids metabolism: a review. Evid Based Complement Alternat Med. 2013; 2013:801457.

[57] Ramírez-Zamora S, Méndez-Rodríguez ML, Olguín-Martínez M, Sánchez-Sevilla L, Quintana-Quintana M, García-García N, Hernández-Muñoz R. Increased erythrocytes by-products of arginine catabolism are associated with hyperglycemia and could be involved in the pathogenesis of type 2 diabetes mellitus. PLoS One. 2013; 8(6):e66823.

[58] Harisa GI. L-Arginine ameliorates arylesterase/ paraoxonase activity of paraoxonase-1 in hypercholesterolemic rats. Asian J Biochem. 2011; 6(3):263–72.

[59] Eligini S, Porro B, Lualdi A, Squellerio I, Veglia F, Chiorino E, Crisci M, Garlaschè A, Giovannardi M, Werba JP, Tremoli E, Cavalca V. Nitric oxide synthetic pathway in red blood cells is impaired in coronary artery disease. PLoS One. 2013; 8(8):e66945.

[60] Palloshi A, Fragasso G, Piatti P, Monti LD, Setola E, Valsecchi G, Galuccio E, Chierchia SL & Margonato A. Effect of oral L -arginine on blood pressure and endothelial function in patients and symptoms with systemic hypertension, Positive exercise tests, and normal coronary arteries. Am J Cardiol. 2004; 93:933–5.

[61] Harisa GI, Mariee AD, Abo-Salem OM, Attia SM. Erythrocyte nitric oxide synthase as a surrogate marker for mercury-induced vascular damage: the modulatory effects of naringin. Environ Toxicol. 2014; 29(11):1314–22.

Chapter 2

Intracellular Cholesterol Lowering as Novel Target for Anti-Atherosclerotic Therapy

Alexander N. Orekhov and Ekaterina A. Ivanova

Additional information is available at the end of the chapter

http://dx.doi.org/10.5772/64363

Abstract

Atherosclerosis and disorders associated with cardiovascular system remain the major problem of modern medicine and the leading cause of mortality in developed countries. According to the current knowledge, atherosclerosis development can begin early in life. Clinically silent early-stage lesions can be detected in a large population of young adults. Despite substantial progress in the recent years, therapy of atherosclerosis mostly remains limited to plasma lipid profile correction. Moreover, no therapy is currently available for the treatment of asymptomatic early stages of the disease. The existing synthetic drugs could not be used for this purpose, because of the unfavourable risk/benefit ratio and high cost of treatment, which has to be long-lasting. In this regard, medications based on natural agents with anti-atherosclerotic activity may offer interesting possibilities. Current research should focus on detection and evaluation of such agents. One of the important tools for anti-atherosclerotic drug evaluation is a cell-based model, which allows measurement of intracellular lipid accumulation. Anti-atherosclerotic activity of various substances can therefore be evaluated by the decrease of intracellular lipid storage. In this chapter, we will discuss the development and application of cellular models based on primary culture of human arterial wall cells that are suitable for detection and measurement of anti-atherosclerotic activity of various substances. Using these models, several natural agents have been successfully evaluated, which led to the development of pharmaceutical products with anti-atherosclerotic activity based on botanicals.

Keywords: atherosclerosis, arteries, cholesterol accumulation, cellular models, anti-atherosclerotic drugs

1. Introduction

Atherosclerosis remains one of the most challenging problems of modern medicine. Epidemiological data on atherosclerosis and cardiovascular diseases are frequently updated and demonstrate an increase in overall mortality, partly because of the ageing of human population, especially in favourable economic conditions [1]. In developed countries, cardiovascular diseases remain the primary cause of overall morbidity and mortality [2]. Atherosclerotic lesions develop in the walls of large arteries and cause occlusion of blood vessels as a result of either arterial wall thickening or thrombus formation on the surface of unstable plaques. This latter condition is especially dangerous, since it can lead to a sudden and often fatal thromboembolia, which represents the first clinical manifestation of atherosclerosis in many patients. By contrast, early stages of the disease usually pass unnoticed. Recent studies have demonstrated that asymptomatic atherosclerosis is, in fact, a widespread condition among young adults [2–5]. In this cohort of subjects, the incidence of atherosclerotic lesions reaches 100%, although no clinical manifestations can be observed [3–5].

The development of atherosclerosis is a complex process, which, despite the significant progress made during the last decade, still remains to be fully understood. Atherosclerosis and related cardiovascular disorders are associated with several known risk factors, including elevated plasma cholesterol level, diabetes, tobacco smoking and others [6, 7].

Modern atherosclerosis prevention strategies are largely based on elimination or attenuation of relevant risk factors, which slows down the atherosclerotic plaque progression in an indirect way [8]. For instance, statins are commonly used for plasma cholesterol reduction and attenuation of atherosclerosis progression. However, limited indications and serious side effects make statins unsuitable for preventive therapy of atherosclerosis, which has to be long-term. Currently, there exists no widespread "direct" anti-atherosclerotic therapy that could be suitable for treatment of the early, subclinical stages of the disease. Such therapy should target the molecular and cellular mechanisms of atherogenesis at the level of blood vessel wall and should result in prevention of *de novo* lesion formation or regression of existing plaques [8–10]. Natural agents appear to be attractive candidates for preventive anti-atherosclerosis therapy because of their favourable safety profile and low cost. Because of their complex composition, biologically active substances of botanical origin and their combinations may have a wider range of effects than synthetic drugs, targeting several atherosclerosis risk factors simultaneously. It is therefore possible that the botanical substances can possess both direct and indirect anti-atherosclerotic effects, such as protective activity at the cellular level combined with cholesterol lowering and hypotensive activity. Current knowledge of cardioprotective effects of natural agents and nutraceuticals is rather limited, although they have been actively studied by several groups during the recent years [11–17]. It is important to establish novel anti-atherosclerotic preventive therapies based on natural products and confirm their effectiveness by clinical studies.

The search for potential anti-atherosclerotic agents and evaluation of their activity requires adequate test models. Lipid accumulation is one of the most prominent features of atherosclerotic lesions. Lipid uptake and storage are performed by several cell types of the arterial wall. Both resident cells and inflammatory cells that are recruited to the lesion site can participate in the process. Increased lipid content can be observed already at the earliest stages of the plaque development. The main source of cholesterol deposit in the arterial wall is low-density lipoprotein (LDL), especially its modified, atherogenic forms. The risk of atherosclerosis development has been demonstrated to be associated with unfavourable plasma lipid profile and the increased contents of atherogenic LDL types, such as small dense LDL [18]. The ability of the blood plasma to cause lipid accumulation in the arterial wall cells is referred to as blood serum atherogenicity [19]. Anti-atherosclerotic effect of a substance can be evaluated by its ability to prevent lipid accumulation in cultured arterial wall cells induced by the exposure to atherogenic LDL. Importantly, lipid profile in cells with or without treatment can precisely be measured to quantitatively evaluate anti-atherosclerotic potential.

In this chapter, we will give an overview of current knowledge on atherosclerotic lesion progression and discuss the development and application of models based on primary culture of human arterial wall cells.

2. Atherosclerotic plaque development

According to the classic lipid theory of atherogenesis, atherosclerotic lesion development is caused by extracellular and intracellular lipid accumulation in the intimal layer of the arterial wall [20, 21]. It has been shown that the major source of lipid accumulation in the intimal cells is circulating LDL, especially its atherogenic forms, such as chemically modified and aggregated LDL. Chemical modification of lipoprotein particles appears to be necessary for the atherogenic effect, since native (non-modified) LDL added to cultured cells could not induce significant lipid accumulation. Atherogenic modifications of LDL in the bloodstream include desialylation, acquisition of negative charge and increase of the particle hydrated density (small dense LDL formation). All these modifications can be accompanied by oxidation [22–25]. Study of the atherogenic LDL modification in the bloodstream currently remains challenging. Different laboratory methods of LDL isolation, quantification and analysis deliver different results, which hinders direct comparison of studies employing different methods and protocols. For instance, analysing LDL size and density by ultracentrifugation in different buffers will give slightly different outcome. Moreover, no consensus has been reached so far on the classification of LDL subfractions [22]. It is likely that LDL particles undergo multiple atherogenic modification in human plasma, but the resulting products are differently evaluated by different methods from several laboratories [26–28]. One of the earliest atherogenic modifications demonstrated to occur in human bloodstream is desialylation. The removal of sialic acid residues from the carbohydrate components of LDL particles is performed by trans-sialidase, which is active in the bloodstream. Increased level of circulating modified LDL leads to aggregation of the particles, which is facilitated by increased surface charge. The resulting large complexes have especially high atherogenic potential. Moreover, modified forms of LDL can induce formation of autoantibodies triggering inflammatory response and giving rise to circulating immune complexes. Another feature that can significantly increase atherogenic potential of modified LDL is its ability to associate with the components of extracellular matrix proteins in the subendothelial space of the arterial wall, which prolongs its residence time and facilitates lipid accumulation. Unlike native LDL, which is internalized by cells via receptor-mediated uptake, modified LDL complexes enter the cells through uncontrolled phagocytosis and follow a distinct metabolic pathway [29]. This can explain the rapid accumulation of atherogenic modified LDL in cellular cytoplasm, mostly in the form of lipid droplets. Cells containing large amounts of lipid inclusions in the cytoplasm are called "foam cells" because of their microscopic appearance. Such cells commonly occur in atherosclerotic lesions.

Figure 1 shows the development of atherosclerotic lesions and the main stages of the atherogenesis [30]. According to the current knowledge, atherosclerotic lesion initiation is dependent on two conditions: the presence of modified atherogenic LDL in the bloodstream in sufficient quantities and the internalization of LDL by the arterial wall cells. The latter is usually triggered by local disturbance of endothelial function that causes increased permeability of the endothelial lining allowing modified LDL to penetrate into the intimal layer of the arterial wall. Atherogenic modification of LDL may also occur in the intimal layer, after the particles have crossed the endothelial barrier. Local disturbances of endothelial function frequently take place in certain parts of the vascular system, such as branching points and bends, where laminar blood flow is altered [31]. Sites of the arterial wall that are especially vulnerable are marked by altered morphology of endothelial cells and presence of enlarged multinucleated cells. The pre-existent mosaicism of the endothelial lining may explain the focal development of atherosclerotic lesions. However, more studies are needed to determine the mechanisms of endothelial dysfunction leading to atherosclerosis.

Focal lipid infiltration into the arterial wall intima marks the early stages of atherosclerotic lesion development. Apparently, several cell types of the arterial wall participate in lipid accumulation. Cells populating the intimal layer can be either resident mesenchymal cells,

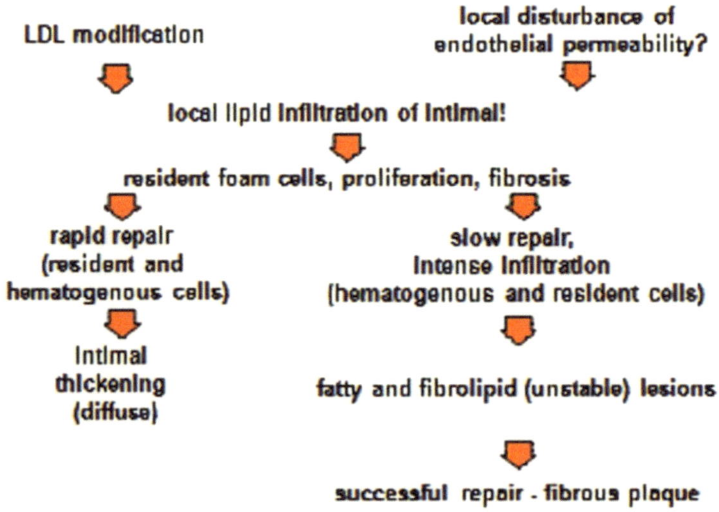

Figure 1. Scheme showing the consecutive events in the development of atherosclerotic lesions. Reproduced with permission from [30].

http://dx.doi.org/10.5772/64363

such as smooth muscle cells, or inflammatory cells, such as monocytes/macrophages, that can be recruited from the bloodstream in large numbers by a local inflammatory response. Along with macrophages, smooth muscular cells also take part in lipid uptake and can be transformed into foam cells. While native LDL particles are metabolized by intimal cells through a well-developed and controlled receptor-mediated endocytosis, it is likely that the LDL associations are recognized by macrophages as pathogens that have to be cleared by phagocytosis [32]. Such clearance is accompanied by secretion of signalling molecules that attract immune cells to the developing lesion site and therefore initiation of the inflammatory process [33]. Phagocytosis-mediated lipid accumulation in atherosclerosis can therefore be regarded as a variation of innate immune response. Enhanced phagocytosis followed by lipid accumulation and foam cell formation contributes to lesion development. Lipid accumulation affects intercellular contacts that are essential for proper function of intimal wall resident cells [34]. On the other hand, lipid accumulation also triggers processes that are typical for the reparative phase of inflammation, such as proliferation and extracellular matrix synthesis leading to the fibrosis. In favourable conditions, these reparation processes rapidly lead to formation of areas with increased cellularity and extracellular matrix deposition. Gradual development of such focal lesion areas leads to a diffuse intimal thickening, which is frequently observed in adult arteries. However, the inflammatory response can become chronic, with continuous local lipid infiltration, increased cellularity due to the proliferation of cells in the lesion site and enhanced fibrosis.

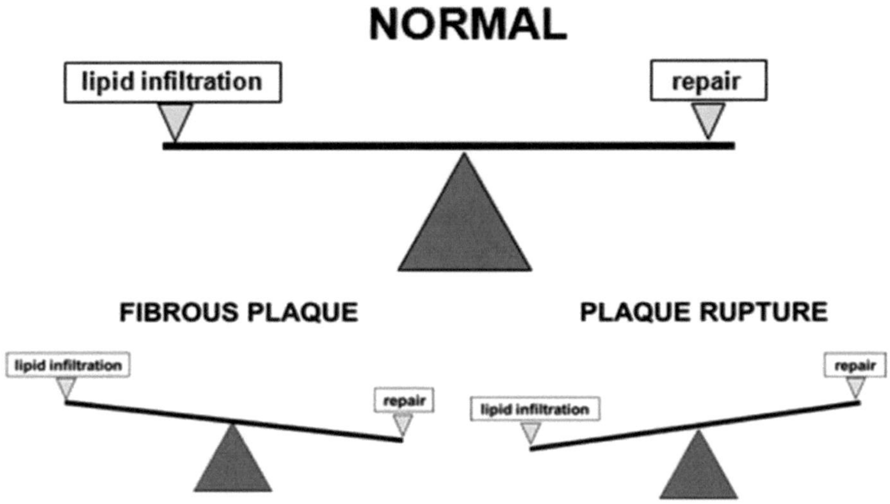

Figure 2. Scheme showing the delicate balance between infiltrative and reparative phases in fatty atherosclerotic lesion. Reproduced with permission from [30].

Atherosclerotic plaques can be protected from the bloodstream by formation of a fibrous cap, which serves as a barrier for lipoproteins and inflammatory cells. Such isolation of the local inflammatory site has a protective role, suppressing the inflammatory response and restoring the tissue functions. On the other hand, formation of fibrolipid plaques predisposed to rupture (unstable plaques) can have fatal consequences because of thrombus formation.

In fibrolipid plaques, two opposing processes are likely to take place: infiltration and reparation that exist in a state of unstable equilibrium (**Figure 2**). Shifting the balance towards reparation leads to the formation of fibrous plaques, which is a favourable outcome from the clinical point of view. Inefficient reparation and continuous lipid infiltration cause plaque rupture with possible thrombus formation. Lipidosis plays therefore a crucial role in atherosclerotic lesion development at cellular and tissue levels and represents an important target for the development of anti-atherosclerotic therapy.

3. Evaluation of substances' anti-atherosclerotic activity using cellular models

Preventive anti-atherosclerotic therapy should be aimed at reduction of intracellular lipid accumulation [35]. Such reduction can be achieved by different approaches [36]. First, the therapy may decrease the level of circulating modified LDL. Second, it can target atherogenic modification of LDL in the bloodstream. Third, it can reduce lipid uptake and storage by the arterial wall cells. Finally, the therapy can be aimed at depletion of the existing intracellular lipid stores. All these approaches can be evaluated by measuring the reduction of intracellular lipid accumulation and the decrease of the intracellular pool of cholesterol esters [9, 37, 38]. A number of available medications can be used to decrease blood serum atherogenicity [9, 36, 38, 39], which is defined as the ability of blood serum to induce cholesterol accumulation in cultured cells. Blood serum from patients with coronary atherosclerosis usually has high atherogenicity [19]. Changes of blood serum atherogenicity reflect lipid accumulation in the arterial wall and are therefore relevant for the development of preventive therapy. Such changes can be detected using cultured cells as models of early stages of human atherogenesis [9, 38, 40]. Cellular models can be used for evaluation of anti-atherosclerotic potential of different drugs and active substances, for screening of potential anti-atherosclerotic agents and for evaluation of potential clinical efficacy of various molecules.

4. *In vitro* model

In vitro model based on primary culture of human aortic wall cells was developed for screening of potential anti-atherosclerotic substances. Cells were isolated from the subendothelial layer of healthy human aortic intima, the layer of the arterial wall, which is most severely affected in atherosclerosis [41]. The process of cell isolation from autopsy material using collagenase and elastase treatment has been described previously [9, 42–44]. The obtained cell population has been characterized using immunocytochemistry methods and was found to be heterogeneous and containing smooth muscle cells (20–50%), pericytes (30–70%) and inflammatory cells and tissue macrophages (10%) (**Table 1**) [9, 43, 44].

Smooth muscle α-actin⁺	3G5⁺	2A7⁺	CD45⁺	CD68⁺
89.6 ± 6.7%	45.8 ± 10.9%	24.1 ± 9.9%	3.6 ± 0.4%	5.2 ± 1.3%

Table 1. Proportion of cell types in primary culture cells isolated from human aortic subendothelial intima (% of positive cells for each marker).

Substance	References
Anti-atherosclerotic	
Cyclic AMP	[9, 44, 46–49]
Prostacyclin	[9, 50–54]
Prostaglandin E_2	[9, 52, 55]
Artificial HDL*	[56]
Antioxidants	[9]
Calcium antagonists	[9, 51, 57–59]
Trapidil and its derivatives	[60, 61]
Lipoxygenase inhibitors	[55]
Lipostabil	[9]
Mushroom extracts	[62]
Pro-atherogenic	
Beta blockers	[58, 63]
Thromboxane A_2	[51, 55]
Phenothiazine	[58]
Indifferent	
Nitrates	[58]
Cholestyramine	[58]
Sulfonylureas	[64]

[a] HDL, high-density lipoprotein.

Table 2. Substances that have been tested *in vitro* cell model.

Smooth muscle cells and pericytes were positive for smooth muscle α-actin. Pericytes had a distinct stellate shape and were identified using antibodies to 3G5 and 2A7 that are expressed by resting and activated pericytes, respectively. Together, smooth muscle cells and pericytes represented the majority of cell population in the obtained primary cultures. A smaller population consisted of the inflammatory cells that could be detected using antibodies to leukocyte-specific marker CD45 and macrophage marker CD68 [45]. Cellular lipid accumulation was induced by incubation of cells with atherogenic serum obtained from patients with confirmed atherosclerosis. The increase of cellular cholesterol content reached as high as two folds after a 24-h incubation with atherogenic serum.

Potential anti-atherogenic substances were evaluated by concomitant incubation of cells with atherogenic serum and aqueous solutions of tested substances. Anti-atherosclerotic effect was measured as a decrease in the levels of intracellular cholesterol in the cells with test substances compared to the control cells (treated with atherogenic serum only). The described model allowed evaluating a number of different drugs and substances and detecting several novel active molecules with anti-atherosclerotic potential. Some substances were demonstrated to possess a pro-atherogenic effect, enhancing intracellular cholesterol accumulation induced by atherogenic serum (**Table 2**).

5. *Ex vivo* model

Ex vivo model is based on primary culture of cells from unaffected human aortic intima that are incubated with blood serum from patients treated with the substance of interest. Therefore, potential anti-atherogenic properties of substances are evaluated based on their pharmacodynamic properties, or the influence on blood serum atherogenicity after digestion and possible metabolic modifications in patient's body. Blood samples are drawn before and after administration of single doses of tested substances, and serum obtained from the samples is added to cultured primary cells. *Ex vivo* model can be used for testing drugs with known safety profiles, as well as various natural products.

Several studies have demonstrated successful application of this model for evaluation of anti-atherogenic properties of botanicals. Screening studies were performed on volunteers (groups of 4–8 men and women 45–60 years old) with high blood serum atherogenicity. One of the tested natural products with anti-atherosclerotic properties was encapsulated onion (*Allium cepa*) bulb powder (300 mg) (**Figure 3**). Administration of a single dose of the product resulted in a moderate decrease of blood serum atherogenicity by 12, 28, and 24% from the baseline after 2, 4, and 6 h, respectively. Another tested natural product with anti-atherosclerotic properties was preparation of wheat seedlings (*Triticum aestivum*). Administration of a single dose of 300 mg of the preparation resulted in a pronounced reduction of blood serum atherogenicity after 4 h (**Figure 4**). Moderate but prolonged anti-atherosclerotic effect was registered for dry beet (*Beta vulgaris*) juice (encapsulated preparation of 300 mg) (**Figure 5**). Garlic (*Allium sativum*) powder possessed a strong and prolonged effect (**Figure 6**). Blood serum atherogenicity was completely suppressed 4 h after administration of a single dose of 300 mg of the preparation. Several other natural products were screened for potential anti-atherosclerotic activity using the *ex vivo* model (**Table 3**). The highest activity after a single dose administration was detected for garlic powder and wheat seedlings, with garlic powder providing the strongest effect. Importantly, anti-atherosclerotic effects of garlic have been reported by several independent groups during the recent years [65–67].

http://dx.doi.org/10.5772/64363

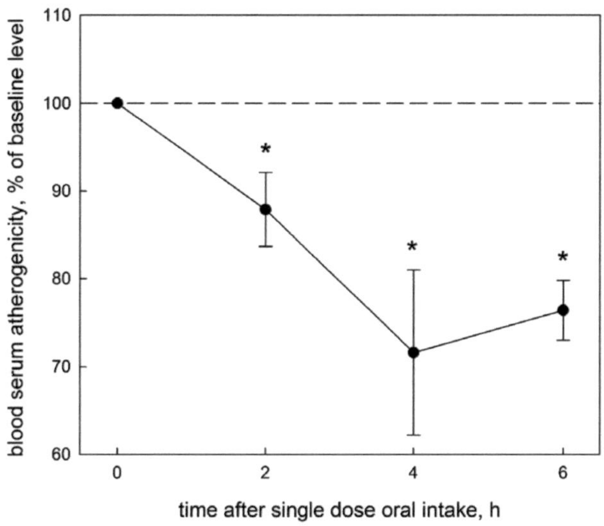

Figure 3. Anti-atherosclerotic effect of onion in *ex vivo* model.The study involved four volunteers (three males, one female, mean age 57 ± 5 years) whose blood serum induced 1.3–1.5-fold increase in cholesterol content of cells cultured from unaffected human aortic intima (the average level of serum atherogenicity was 141 ± 4%). Intracellular cholesterol in control cultures was 38.4 ± 1.1 mg/mg cell protein. Baseline serum atherogenicity was taken as 100%. The average values of changes of serum atherogenicity with indication of standard errors are presented. Reproduced with permission from [30].

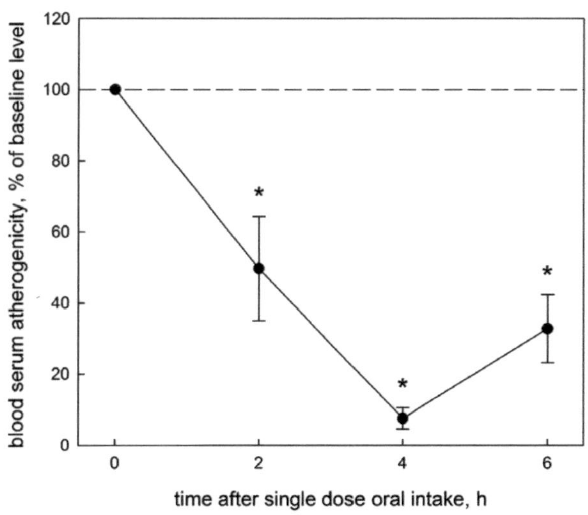

Figure 4. Anti-atherosclerotic effect of wheat seedlings in *ex vivo* model.The study involved eight volunteers (five males, three females, mean age 51 ± 2 years) whose blood serum induced 1.7–2.3-fold increase in cholesterol content of cells cultured from unaffected human aortic intima (the average level of serum atherogenicity was 199 ± 6%). Intracellular cholesterol in control cultures was 28.0 ± 1.2 mg/mg cell protein. Baseline serum atherogenicity was taken as 100%. The average values of changes of serum atherogenicity with indication of standard errors are presented. *, Significant decrease of serum atherogenicity, $p < 0.05$. Reproduced with permission from [30].

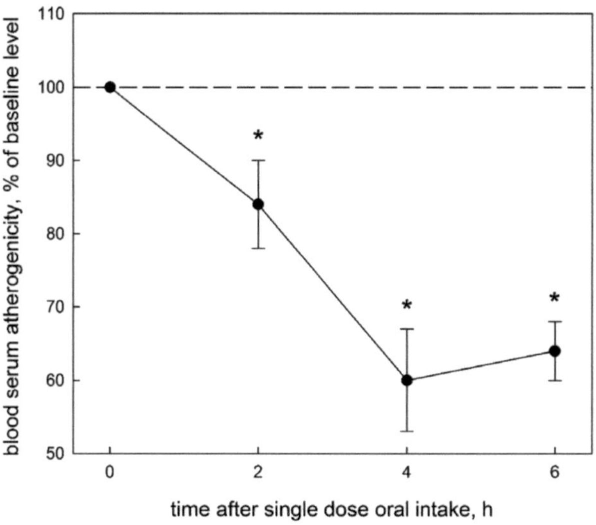

Figure 5. Anti-atherosclerotic effect of beet juice in *ex vivo* model.The study involved eight volunteers (six males, two females, mean age 53 ± 5 years) whose blood serum induced 1.3–2.2-fold increase in cholesterol content of cells cultured from unaffected human aortic intima (the average level of serum atherogenicity was 161 ± 8%). Intracellular cholesterol in control cultures was 37.0 ± 3.6 mg/mg cell protein. Baseline serum atherogenicity was taken as 100%. The average values of changes of serum atherogenicity with indication of standard errors are presented. *, Significant decrease of serum atherogenicity, $p < 0.05$. Reproduced with permission from [30].

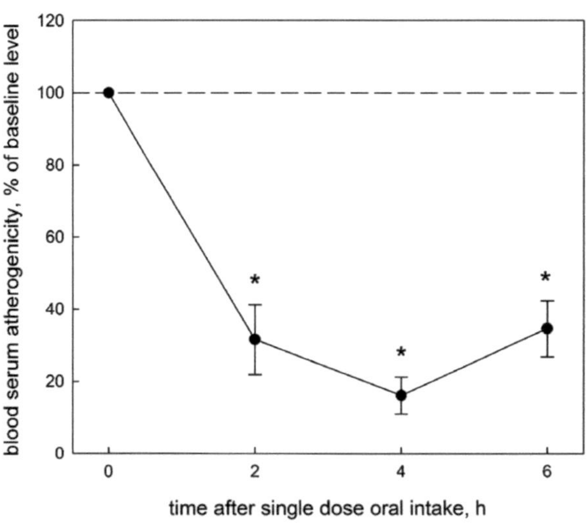

Figure 6. Anti-atherosclerotic effect of garlic powder in the *ex vivo* model.The study involved eight volunteers (six males, two females, mean age 53 ± 5 years) whose blood serum induced 1.3–2.7-fold increase in cholesterol content of cells cultured from unaffected human aortic intima (the average level of serum atherogenicity was 164 ± 9%). Intracellular cholesterol in control cultures was 39.0 ± 4.2 mg/mg cell protein. Baseline serum atherogenicity was taken as 100%. The average values of changes of serum atherogenicity with indication of standard errors are presented. *, Significant decrease of serum atherogenicity, $p < 0.05$. Reproduced with permission from [30].

Botanical and its source	The mean efficiency of atherogenic reduction (%)	Maximum effect (%)
Spirulina platensis powder	50.7	61
Onion (*Allium cepa*) bulb powder	21.4	28
Beet (*Beta vulgaris*) juice powder	30.7	40
Wheat (*Triticum vulgaris*) seedlings powder	70.0	100
Licorice (*Glycyrrhiza glabra*) root powder	54.6	32
Salsola collina leaf powder	10.9	28
Garlic (*Allium sativum*) bulbs powder	76.6	100
Pine (*Pinus sylvestris*) needles extract	52.1	62

*The integrated effect was calculated as a mean reduction in serum atherogenicity for 6 h after a single oral dose.

Table 3. Integral estimation of anti-atherogenic actions of natural products*.

The described *ex vivo* model could be used for establishing the effective dose and posology of the potential anti-atherosclerotic natural products. For this purpose, blood samples were drawn before and after (2 and 4 h) administration of a single dose to patients with high blood serum atherogenicity. Dose dependency was tested by comparison of the effect of two different doses. Each dose was evaluated on at least six different study participants. It was demonstrated that the anti-atherosclerotic effect of garlic powder was present in the dose range from 50 to 300 mg with half-maximal effect observed at a dose of 100 mg, and maximal effect—at 150 mg. Therefore, natural products of botanical origin can be regarded as an important source of agents with anti-atherosclerotic activity that can be used for the development of direct anti-atherosclerotic therapy. Based on the obtained results, several dietary supplements were registered and further evaluated in clinical studies presented below.

As any model, cellular models for studying atherosclerosis development have their limitations [68–71]. Limitations of the experimental models used for atherosclerosis research have been discussed in a number of comprehensive reviews [72–77]. However, the described test system allows performing the initial screening for anti-atherosclerotic activity that can be further studied and confirmed in pre-clinical and clinical studies.

6. Clinical studies

Tests on cellular models demonstrated that garlic powder preparations possessed a pronounced anti-atherosclerotic activity. Based on the obtained results, a garlic-based dietary supplement (Allicor, INAT-Farma, Russia) was developed. The effect of the supplement on carotid intima-media thickness (cIMT) was evaluated in an open-label prospective pilot study conducted on 28 men (46–58 years old, mean age 52.0, SD = 9.0). The study participants had no signs of coronary heart disease, no chronic diseases requiring treatment with vasoactive drugs, diuretics, lipid-lowering or antidiabetic drugs and were normolipidemic or mildly hyperlipidemic. Study subjects were analysed for presence of diffuse intimal thickening by ultrasound imaging of common carotid arteries [65]. The cut-off cIMT value of 0.7 mm in the distal segment of at least one common carotid artery was set up to diagnose diffuse intimal thickening. The mean cIMT value at the baseline was 0.832 ± 0.024 mm. Study participants were divided into two groups. Subjects from Allicor group (n = 16) received 600 mg of Allicor daily, and subjects from the control group (n = 12) received no treatment. The total duration of the study was 12 months, with interviews and ultrasound assessment of cIMT every 3 months. No adverse effects were observed during the follow-up period, and the product was demonstrated to have good tolerability. The results of cIMT assessments are presented on **Figure 7**.

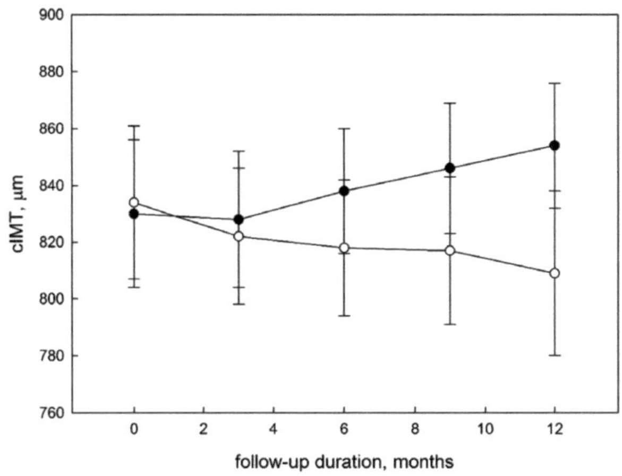

Figure 7. The effects of garlic-based drug Allicor on atherosclerosis determined by cIMT. Open circles, Allicor recipients; solid circles, control subjects. Presented are mean values ±S.E.M. Reproduced from [30].

No statistically significant changes of cIMT were observed after 12 months, and the value was not significantly different between the two groups. However, regression analysis revealed a significant difference between the trends of cIMT dynamics ($p < 0.05$). In the control group, a tendency to cIMT increase was detected, which was significantly different from that of null hypothesis of no change (F-test, 31.72; $p = 0.011$). In the Allicor-treated group, the tendency to cIMT decrease was revealed, which was also significantly different from that of null hypothesis (F-test, 28.81; $p = 0.013$). These results indicate that treatment with Allicor may potentially halter the development and induce the regression of subclinical atherosclerosis. The statistical power of this pilot study was insufficient to avoid type 2 error. Therefore, the pilot study was followed by a larger prospective clinical study, in which a number of clinical and biochemical parameters associated with atherogenesis were taken into account. The dynamic of serum atherogenicity was also assessed. This double-blind placebo-controlled clinical study evaluated the effect of garlic powder tablets Allicor on the progression of cIMT in 211 men (40–74 years old) with no symptoms of atherosclerosis (ClinicalTrials.gov identifier, NCT01734707). The primary outcome was the progression of subclinical atherosclerosis evaluated by B-mode ultrasonography as the increase of cIMT. By the end of the first 12-month follow-up period, a decrease of cIMT by 0.028 ± 0.008 mm was observed in the Allicor group. At the same time, moderate increase of 0.014 ± 0.009 mm was observed in the placebo group ($p = 0.002$). Serum atherogenicity was decreased in the Allicor group by 45% from the baseline and remained unaltered in the placebo group. Therefore, long-term treatment with Allicor had a direct anti-atherosclerotic effect in patients with subclinical atherosclerosis associated with decreased serum atherogenicity [78]. By the end of the 24-month follow-up period, the mean rate of cIMT was decreased in the Allicor group by 0.022 ± 0.007 mm per year, which was significantly different ($p = 0.002$) from the placebo group, in which there was a moderate but statistically significant progression of 0.015 ± 0.008 mm at the overall mean baseline cIMT of 0.931 ± 0.009 mm [37, 39]. A significant reduction of cIMT was observed in 47.3% of study subjects from the Allicor group vs 30.1% in the placebo group ($p < 0.05$). Further significant increase of cIMT was registered in 32.2% study participants in Allicor-treated group vs 47.3% in placebo group ($p < 0.05$). Study of blood serum atherogenicity demonstrated a 1.56-fold increase of intracellular cholesterol accumulation in the cellular test at the baseline. Study participants from Allicor group had an average 30% decrease of blood serum atherogenicity, while in the placebo group, this parameter remained unaltered during the study. A significant correlation was observed between changes of blood serum atherogenicity and intima-media thickness of common carotid arteries ($r = 0.144$, $p = 0.045$) (**Figures 8** and **9**). Therefore, it was demonstrated that garlic-based food supplement Allicor possessed a direct anti-atherosclerotic effect at the subclinical stage of the disease, which could be attributed to the decrease of blood serum atherogenicity [37, 39].

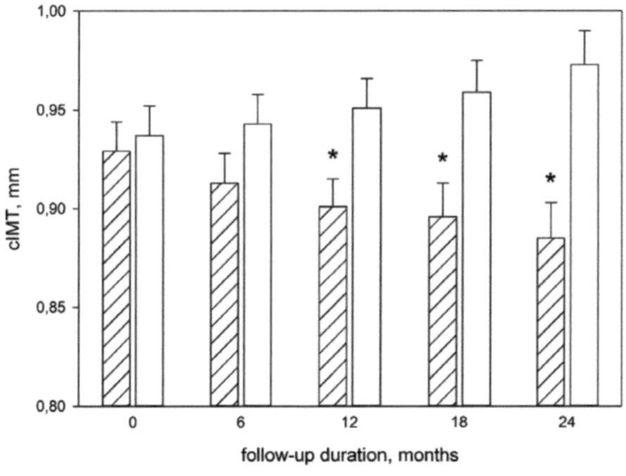

Figure 8. The dynamics of cIMT in double-blind placebo-controlled study on anti-atherosclerotic effects of garlic-based drug Allicor. Hatched bars, Allicor recipients; open bars, placebo recipients. Presented are mean values ±S.E.M. *, significant difference between groups, $p < 0.05$. Reproduced with permission from [30].

Another clinical study was focused on the evaluation of potential anti-atherosclerotic activity of herbal products with anti–inflammatory effects. Atherosclerosis is tightly associated with the inflammatory process at all stages of the disease development [79, 80]. Substances with systemic anti-inflammatory properties can therefore be regarded as potential therapeutic agents for treatment and prevention of atherosclerosis.

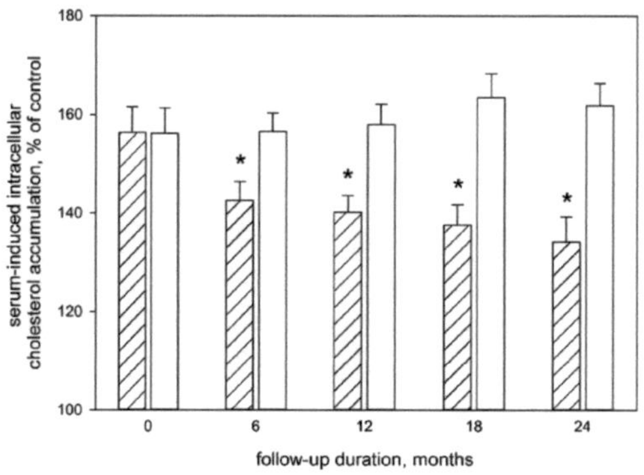

Figure 9. The dynamics of serum atherogenicity in double-blind placebo-controlled study on anti-atherosclerotic effects of garlic-based drug Allicor. Hatched bars, Allicor recipients; open bars, placebo recipients. Presented are mean values ±S.E.M. *, significant difference between groups, $p < 0.05$. Reproduced with permission from [30].

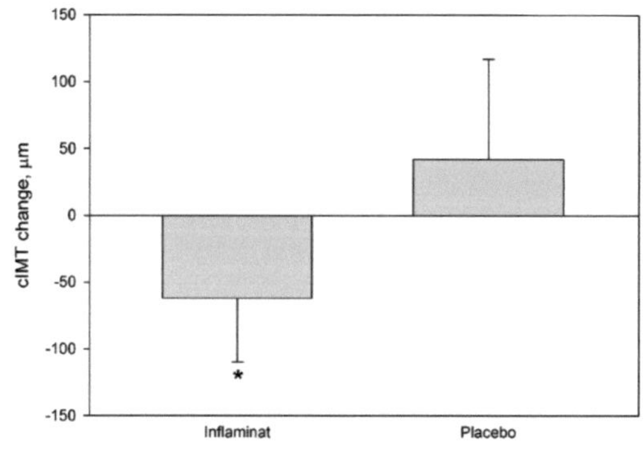

Figure 10. The changes of cIMT in double-masked placebo-controlled study on anti-atherosclerotic effects of Inflaminat. Presented are mean values ±S.E.M. *, significant difference between groups, $p < 0.05$. Reproduced with permission from [30].

Several natural compounds, such as calendula (*Calendula officinalis*), elder (*Sambucus nigra*) and violet (*Viola* sp.), were demonstrated to possess not only anti-inflammatory, but also anti-atherosclerotic effects [81–83]. The combination of these herbs was used for the development of a novel dietary supplement (Inflaminat, INAT-Farma, Russia) [84]. The effect of Inflaminat on cIMT dynamics was evaluated in a pilot placebo-controlled double-blinded study performed on 67 asymptomatic men (ClinicalTrials.gov Identifier, NCT01743404) [39, 85]. The protocol of the 12-month study was similar to that described for Allicor food supplement. Administration of Inflaminat induced cIMT regression in subclinical atherosclerosis, with statistically significant difference between the baseline as the placebo group (**Figure 10**). Therefore, Inflaminat was demonstrated to possess anti-inflammatory and anti-atherosclerotic effects at the cellular level and to induce regression of subclinical atherosclerotic lesions in asymptomatic men.

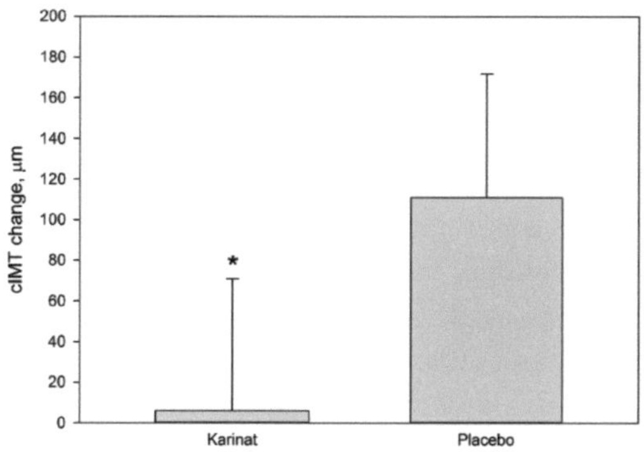

Figure 11. The changes of cIMT in double-masked placebo-controlled study on anti-atherosclerotic effects of Karinat. The data are presented in the terms of means and S.D. *, significant difference between groups, $p < 0.05$. Reproduced with permission from [30].

Finally, several phytoestrogen-rich natural substances were evaluated for potential anti-atherosclerotic activity using the described *in vitro* and an *ex vivo* models [86–88]. The most promising of these compounds were garlic powder, extract of grape seeds, green tea leaf and hop cones. All these substances possessed a significant anti-atherogenic effect. A combination of these compounds was used for development of a novel isoflavonoid-rich dietary supplement (Karinat, INAT-Farma, Russia). The resulting supplement is a source of biologically active polyphenols, including resveratrol, genisteine and daidzeine that are claimed to produce beneficial effects on atherosclerosis development. The efficiency of Karinat was evaluated in a randomized double-blind placebo-controlled 12-month clinical study conducted on 157 asymptomatic postmenopausal women (ClinicalTrials.gov Identifier, NCT01742000) [89, 90]. The primary endpoint was the annual rate of cIMT change. The protocol of the study was similar to that reported above. An annual increase of mean cIMT of more than 100 µm (13% per year) was observed in the placebo group, indicative of a high rate of cIMT progression in postmenopausal women. Growth of atherosclerotic plaques was estimated to be 40% per year. In the Karinat group, mean cIMT value remained unaltered, with a statistically insignificant increase of 6 µm per year, *that is* <1% (**Figure 11**). Therefore, phytoestrogen-rich substances were proven to possess beneficial effects on the dynamics of subclinical atherosclerosis progression in postmenopausal women [39, 91].

7. Conclusions

Introduction of the concept of blood serum atherogenicity allowed creating cell model suitable for screening of substances with potential anti-atherosclerotic activity. Such models helped revealing several novel compounds of botanical origin that could be used for the development of dietary supplements for treatment of subclinical (asymptomatic) atherosclerosis. The effect of "direct" anti-atherosclerotic therapy can be observed at the level of the arterial wall cells by a decrease of intracellular lipid accumulation. Therapy of patients with established atherosclerosis should induce regression of the existing plaques or hinder the progression of novel lesions. Introduction of food supplements from botanicals with anti-atherosclerotic properties and suitable for long-term consumption is an important step toward the improvement of the preventive treatment of atherosclerosis. Further studies will help revealing natural products with anti-atherogenic and anti-atherosclerotic effects that can be used for the development of novel cardiovascular drugs possessing mechanistic mode of action. Despite the unavoidable limitations of the described models, the obtained results have demonstrated that cultured arterial wall cells offer a suitable instrument for initial analysis of drug effects. The discovery of anti-atherosclerotic activity of natural products opens great opportunities for prevention and treatment of atherosclerotic disease, reducing cardiovascular morbidity and mortality.

Disclosure statement

The authors report no conflict of interest.

Acknowledgements

The work was supported by Ministry of Education and Sciences, Russia (Project # RFMEFI61614X0010).

Author details

Alexander N. Orekhov[1,2,3] and Ekaterina A. Ivanova[4*]

*Address all correspondence to: kate.ivanov@gmail.com

1 Department of Biophysics, Faculty of Biology, Lomonosov Moscow State University, Moscow, Russia

2 Laboratory of Angiopathology, Institute of General Pathology and Pathophysiology, Moscow, Russia

3 Institute for Atherosclerosis Research, Skolkovo Innovative Center, Moscow, Russia

4 KU Leuven, Department of Development and Regeneration, Leuven, Belgium

References

[1] Barquera S, Pedroza-Tobias A, Medina C, Hernandez-Barrera L, Bibbins-Domingo K, Lozano R, Moran AE. Global overview of the epidemiology of atherosclerotic cardiovascular disease. Arch Med Res 2015; 46: 328–38.

[2] Simmons A, Steffen K, Sanders S. Medical therapy for peripheral arterial disease. Curr Opin Cardiol 2012; 27: 592–7.

[3] Berenson GS, Srinivasan SR, Bao W, Newman WP 3rd, Tracy RE, Wattigney WA. Association between multiple cardiovascular risk factors and atherosclerosis in children and young adults. The Bogalusa Heart Study. N Engl J Med 1998; 338: 1650–6.

[4] McGill HC Jr, Herderick EE, McMahan CA, Zieske AW, Malcolm GT, Tracy RE, Strong JP. Atherosclerosis in youth. Minerva Pediatr 2002; 54: 437–47.

[5] Tuzcu EM, Kapadia SR, Tutar E, Ziada KM, Hobbs RE, McCarthy PM, Young JB, Nissen SE. High prevalence of coronary atherosclerosis in asymptomatic teenagers and young adults: evidence from intravascular ultrasound. Circulation 2001; 103: 2705–10.

[6] Anderson KM, Wilson PW, Odell PM, Kannel WB. An updated coronary risk profile. A statement for health professionals. Circulation 1991; 83: 356–62.

[7] Fowkes FG, Rudan D, Rudan I, Aboyans V, Denenberg JO, McDermott MM, Norman PE, Sampson UK, Williams LJ, Mensah GA, Criqui MH. Comparison of global estimates of prevalence and risk factors for peripheral artery disease in 2000 and 2010: a systematic review and analysis. Lancet 2013; 382: 1329–40.

[8] Orekhov AN, Tertov VV. *In vitro* effect of garlic powder extract on lipid content in normal and atherosclerotic human aortic cells. Lipids 1997; 32: 1055–60.

[9] Orekhov AN, Tertov VV, Kudryashov SA, Khashimov KhA, Smirnov VN. Primary culture of human aortic intima cells as a model for testing antiatherosclerotic drugs. Effects of cyclic AMP, prostaglandins, calcium antagonists, antioxidants, and lipid-lowering agents. Atherosclerosis 1986; 60: 101–10.

[10] Sazonova M, Budnikov E, Khasanova Z, Sobenin I, Postnov A, Orekhov A. Studies of the human aortic intima by a direct quantitative assay of mutant alleles in the mitochondrial genome. Atherosclerosis 2009; 204: 184–90.

[11] Rai AK, Debetto P, Sala FD. Molecular regulation of cholesterol metabolism: HDL-based intervention through drugs and diet. Indian J Exp Biol 2013; 51: 885–94.

[12] Al-Waili N, Salom K, Al-Ghamdi A, Ansari MJ, Al-Waili A, Al-Waili T. Honey and cardiovascular risk factors, in normal individuals and in patients with diabetes mellitus or dyslipidemia. J Med Food 2013; 16: 1063–78.

[13] Ried K, Toben C, Fakler P. Effect of garlic on serum lipids: an updated meta-analysis. Nutr Rev 2013; 71: 282–99.

[14] Hopkins AL, Lamm MG, Funk JL, Ritenbaugh C. Hibiscus sabdariffa L. In the treatment of hypertension and hyperlipidemia: a comprehensive review of animal and human studies. Fitoterapia 2013; 85: 84–94.

[15] Sobenin IA, Nedosugova LV, Filatova LV, Balabolkin MI, Gorchakova TV, Orekhov AN. Metabolic effects of time-released garlic powder tablets in type 2 diabetes mellitus: the results of double-blinded placebo-controlled study. Acta Diabetol 2008; 45: 1–6.

[16] Sobenin IA, Pryanishnikov VV, Kunnova LM, Rabinovich YA, Martirosyan DM, Orekhov AN. The effects of time-released garlic powder tablets on multifunctional cardiovascular risk in patients with coronary artery disease. Lipids Health Dis 2010; 9: 119.

[17] Sobenin IA, Andrianova IV, Fomchenkov IV, Gorchakova TV, Orekhov AN. Time-released garlic powder tablets lower systolic and diastolic blood pressure in men with mild and moderate arterial hypertension. Hypertens Res 2009; 32: 433–7.

[18] Diffenderfer MR, Schaefer EJ. The composition and metabolism of large and small LDL. Curr Opin Lipidol. 2014; 25: 221–6.

[19] Chazov EI, Tertov VV, Orekhov AN, Lyakishev AA, Perova NV, Kurdanov KA, Khashimov KA, Novikov ID, Smirnov VN. Atherogenicity of blood serum from patients with coronary heart disease. Lancet 1986; 2: 595–8.

[20] Schönfelder M. Ortologie und patologie der Langhans-zellen der aortenintima des menschen. Pathol Microbiol (Basel) 1969; 33: 129–45.

[21] Konstantinov IE, Mejevoi N, Anichkov NM. Nikolai N. Anichkov and his theory of atherosclerosis. Tex Heart Inst J 2006; 33: 417–23.

[22] Jaakkola O, Solakivi T, Tertov VV, Orekhov AN, Miettinen TA, Nikkari T. Characteristics of low-density lipoprotein subfractions from patients with coronary artery disease. Coron Artery Dis 1993; 4: 379–85.

[23] Sobenin IA, Tertov VV, Orekhov AN. Optimization of the assay for sialic acid determination in low density lipoprotein. J Lipid Res 1998; 39: 2293–9.

[24] Tertov VV, Sobenin IA, Gabbasov ZA, Popov EG, Jaakkola O, Solakivi T, Nikkari T, Smirnov VN, Orekhov AN. Multiple-modified desialylated low density lipoproteins that cause intracellular lipid accumulation. Isolation, fractionation and characterization. Lab Invest 1992; 67: 665–75.

[25] Tertov VV, Sobenin IA, Orekhov AN. Modified (desialylated) low-density lipoprotein measured in serum by lectin-sorbent assay. Clin Chem 1995; 41: 1018–21.

[26] Tertov VV, Bittolo-Bon G, Sobenin IA, Cazzolato G, Orekhov AN, Avogaro P. Naturally occurring modified low density lipoproteins are similar if not identical: more electronegative and desialylated lipoprotein subfractions. Exp Mol Pathol 1995; 62: 166–72.

[27] Tertov VV, Sobenin IA, Orekhov AN. Similarity between naturally occurring modified desialylated, electronegative and aortic low density lipoprotein. Free Radic Res 1996; 25: 313–319.

[28] Tertov VV, Sobenin IA, Gabbasov ZA, Popov EG, Yaroslavov AA, Jauhiainen M, Ehnholm C, Smirnov VN, Orekhov AN. Three types of naturally occurring modified lipoproteins induce intracellular lipid accumulation in human aortic intimal cells – the role of lipoprotein aggregation. Eur J Clin Chem Clin Biochem 1992; 30: 171–8.

[29] Goldstein JL, Brown MS. Regulation of low-density lipoprotein receptors: implications for pathogenesis and therapy of hypercholesterolemia and atherosclerosis. Circulation 1987; 76: 504–7.

[30] Orekhov AN, Sobenin IA, Revin VV, Bobryshev YV. Development of antiatherosclerotic drugs on the basis of natural products using cell model approach. Oxid Med Cell Longev 2015; 2015: 46379, doi:10.1155/2015/463797.

[31] Vanhoutte PM. How we learned to say NO. Arterioscler Thromb Vasc Biol. 2009; 29: 1156–1160.

[32] Kruth HS. Sequestration of aggregated low-density lipoproteins by macrophages. Curr Opin Lipidol. 2002; 13: 483–488.

[33] Gratchev A, Sobenin I, Orekhov A, Kzhyshkowska J. Monocytes as a diagnostic marker of cardiovascular diseases. Immunobiology 2012; 217: 476–82.

[34] Andreeva ER, Pugach IM, Orekhov AN. Collagen-synthesizing cells in initial and advanced atherosclerotic lesions of human aorta. Atherosclerosis 1997; 130: 133–42.

[35] Orekhov AN, Andreeva ER, Bobryshev YV. Cellular mechanisms of human atherosclerosis: role of cell-to-cell communications in subendothelial cell functions. Tissue Cell. 2016; 48: 25–34.

[36] Orekhov AN. Direct anti-atherosclerotic therapy; development of natural anti-atherosclerotic drugs preventing cellular cholesterol retention. Curr Pharm Des 2013; 19: 5909–28.

[37] Sobenin IA, Chistiakov DA, Bobryshev YV, Orekhov AN. Blood atherogenicity as a target for anti-atherosclerotic therapy. Curr Pharm Des 2013; 19: 5954–5962.

[38] Orekhov AN, Tertov VV, Lyakishev AA, Ruda MY. Use of cultured atherosclerotic cells for investigation of antiatherosclerotic effects of anipamil and other calcium antagonists. J Hum Hypertens. 1991; 5: 425–430.

[39] Orekhov AN, Sobenin IA, Korneev NV, Kirichenko TV, Myasoedova VA, Melnichenko AA, Balcells M, Edelman ER, Bobryshev YV. Anti-atherosclerotic therapy based on botanicals. Recent Pat Cardiovasc Drug Discov 2013; 8: 56–66.

[40] Orekhov AN, Tertov VV, Kudryashov SA, Smirnov VN. Triggerlike stimulation of cholesterol accumulation and DNA and extracellular matrix synthesis induced by atherogenic serum or low density lipoprotein in cultured cells. Circ Res 1990; 66: 311–320.

[41] Rekhter MD, Andreeva ER, Mironov AA, Orekhov AN. Three-dimensional cytoarchitecture of normal and atherosclerotic intima of human aorta. Am J Pathol 1991; 138: 569–580.

[42] Orekhov AN, Andreeva ER, Krushinsky AV, Smirnov VN. Primary cultures of enzyme-isolated cells from normal and atherosclerotic human aorta. Med Biol 1984; 62: 255–259.

[43] Orekhov AN, Tertov VV, Novikov ID, Krushinsky AV, Andreeva ER, Lankin VZ, Smirnov VN. Lipids in cells of atherosclerotic and uninvolved human aorta. I. Lipid composition of aortic tissue and enzyme-isolated and cultured cells. Exp Mol Pathol 1985; 42: 117–137.

[44] Orekhov AN, Krushinsky AV, Andreeva ER, Repin VS, Smirnov VN. Adult human aortic cells in primary culture: heterogeneity in shape. Heart Vessels 1986; 2: 193–201.

[45] Andreeva ER, Pugach IM, Orekhov AN. Subendothelial smooth muscle cells of human aorta express macrophage antigen *in situ* and *in vitro*. Atherosclerosis. 1997; 135: 19–27.

[46] Tertov VV, Orekhov AN, Repin VS, Smirnov VN. Dibutyryl cyclic AMP decrease proliferative activity and the cholesteryl ester content in cultured cells of atherosclerotic human aorta. Biochem Biophys Res Commun 1982; 109: 1228–33.

[47] Tertov VV, Orekhov AN, Smirnov VN. Agents that increase cellular cyclic AMP inhibit proliferative activity and decrease lipid content in cells cultured from atherosclerotic human aorta. Artery 1986; 13: 365–372.

[48] Tertov VV, Orekhov AN, Smirnov VN. Effect of cyclic AMP on lipid accumulation and metabolism in human atherosclerotic aortic cells. Atherosclerosis 1986; 62: 55–64.

[49] Tertov VV, Orekhov AN, Grigorian GYu, Kurennaya GS, Kudryashov SA, Tkachuk VA, Smirnov VN. Disorders in the system of cyclic nucleotides in atherosclerosis: cyclic

AMP and cyclic GMP content and activity of related enzymes in human aorta. Tissue Cell 1987; 19: 21–28.

[50] Akopov SE, Orekhov AN, Tertov VV, Khashimov KA, Gabrielyan ES, Smirnov VN. Stable analogues of prostacyclin and thromboxane A2 display contradictory influences on atherosclerotic properties of cells cultured from human aorta. The effect of calcium antagonists. Atherosclerosis 1988; 72: 245–248.

[51] Baldenkov GN, Akopov SE, Ryong LH, Orekhov AN. Prostacyclin, thromboxane A2 and calcium antagonists: effects on atherosclerotic characteristics of vascular cells. Biomed Biochim Acta 1988; 47: S324–327.

[52] Kudryashov SA, Tertov VV, Orekhov AN, Geling NG, Smirnov VN. Regression of atherosclerotic manifestations in primary culture of human aortic cells: effects of prostaglandins. Biomed Biochim Acta 1984; 43: S284–286.

[53] Orekhov AN, Tertov VV, Smirnov VN. Prostacyclin analogues as anti-atherosclerotic drugs. Lancet 1983; 2: 521.

[54] Orekhov AN, Tertov VV, Mazurov AV, Andreeva ER, Repin VS, Smirnov VN. "Regression" of atherosclerosis in cell culture: effects of stable prostacyclin analogues. Drug Develop Res 1986; 9: 189–201.

[55] Tertov VV, Panosyan AG, Akopov SE, Orekhov AN. The effects of eicozanoids and lipoxygenase inhibitors on the lipid metabolism of aortic cells. Biomed Biochim Acta 1988; 47: S286–288.

[56] Orekhov AN, Misharin AYu, Tertov VV, Khashimov KhA, Pokrovsky SN, Repin VS, Smirnov VN. Artificial HDL as an anti-atherosclerotic drug. Lancet 1984; 2: 1149–1150.

[57] Orekhov AN, Tertov VV, Khashimov KA, Kudryashov SS, Smirnov VN. Evidence of antiatherosclerotic action of verapamil from direct effects on arterial cells. Am J Cardiol 1987; 59: 495–496.

[58] Orekhov AN, Baldenkov GN, Tertov VV, Ryong LH, Kozlov SG, Lyakishev AA, Tkachuk VA, Ruda MYa, Smirnov VN. Cardiovascular drugs and atherosclerosis: effects of calcium antagonists, beta-blockers, and nitrates on atherosclerotic characteristics of human aortic cells. J Cardiovasc Pharmacol 1988; 12 (Suppl 6): S66–68.

[59] Orekhov AN, Baldenkov GN, Tertov VV, Ruda MYa, Khashimov KA, Kudryashov SA, Ryong LH, Kozlov SG, Lyakishev AA, Tkachuk VA, Smirnov VN. Antiatherosclerotic effects of calcium antagonists. Study in human aortic cell culture. Herz 1990; 15: 139–145.

[60] Giessler C, Fahr A, Tertov VV, Kudryashov SA, Orekhov AN, Smirnov VN, Mest HJ. Trapidil derivatives as potential anti-atherosclerotic drugs. Arzneimittelforschung 1987; 37: 538–541.

[61] Heinroth-Hoffmann I, Kruger J, Tertov VV, Orekhov AN, Mest HJ. Influence of trapidil and trapidil derivatives on the content of cyclic nucleotides in human intima cells cultured from atherosclerotic plaques. Drug Develop Res 1990; 19: 321–327.

[62] Li HR, Tertov VV, Vasil'ev AV, Tutel'yan VA, Orekhov AN. Anti-atherogenic and antiatherosclerotic effects of mushroom extracts revealed in human aortic intima cell culture. Drug Develop Res 1989; 17: 109–117.

[63] Orekhov AN, Ruda MYa, Baldenkov GN, Tertov VV, Khashimov KA, Ryong LH, Lyakishev AA, Kozlov SG, Tkachuk VA, Smirnov VN. Atherogenic effects of beta blockers on cells cultured from normal and atherosclerotic aorta. Am J Cardiol 1988; 61: 1116–1117.

[64] Sobenin IA, Maksumova MA, Slavina ES, Balabolkin MI, Orekhov AN. Sulfonylureas induce cholesterol accumulation in cultured human intimal cells and macrophages. Atherosclerosis 1994; 105: 159–163.

[65] Karagodin VP, Sobenin IA, Orekhov AN. Antiatherosclerotic and cardioprotective effects of time-released garlic powder pills. Curr Pharm Des. 2015; 22: 196–213.

[66] Sung J, Harfouche Y, De La Cruz M, Zamora MP, Liu Y, Rego JA, Buckley NE. Garlic (*Allium sativum*) stimulates lipopolysaccharide-induced tumor necrosis factor-alpha production from J774A.1 murine macrophages. Phytother Res. 2015; 29: 288–294.

[67] Koscielny J, Klüssendorf D, Latza R, Schmitt R, Radtke H, Siegel G, Kiesewetter H. The antiatherosclerotic effect of *Allium sativum*. Atherosclerosis. 1999; 144: 237–249.

[68] Hartung T, Daston G. Are *in vitro* tests suitable for regulatory use? Toxicol Sci 2009; 111: 233–237.

[69] Hill BT. *In vitro* human tumour model systems for investigating drug resistance. Cancer Surv 1986; 5: 129–149.

[70] Camenisch G, Folkers G, van de Waterbeemd H. Review of theoretical passive drug absorption models: historical background, recent developments and limitations. Pharm Acta Helv 1996; 71: 309–327.

[71] Bocan TM. Animal models of atherosclerosis and interpretation of drug intervention studies. Curr Pharm Des 1998; 4: 37–52.

[72] Carmeliet P, Moons L, Collen D. Mouse models of angiogenesis, arterial stenosis, atherosclerosis and hemostasis. Cardiovasc Res 1998; 39: 8–33.

[73] Johnson GJ, Griggs TR, Badimon L. The utility of animal models in the preclinical study of interventions to prevent human coronary artery restenosis: analysis and recommendations. On behalf of the Subcommittee on Animal, Cellular and Molecular Models of Thrombosis and Haemostasis of the Scientific and Standardization Committee of the

International Society on Thrombosis and Haemostasis. Thromb Haemost 1999; 81: 835–843.

[74] Moghadasian MH, Frohlich JJ, McManus BM. Advances in experimental dyslipidemia and atherosclerosis. Lab Invest 2001; 81: 1173–1183.

[75] Kones R. Primary prevention of coronary heart disease: integration of new data, evolving views, revised goals, and role of rosuvastatin in management. A comprehensive survey. Drug Des Devel Ther 2011; 5: 325–380.

[76] Peng X. Transgenic rabbit models for studying human cardiovascular diseases. Comp Med 2012; 62: 472–479.

[77] Getz GS, Reardon CA. Animal models of atherosclerosis. Arterioscler Thromb Vasc Biol. 2012; 32: 1104–1115.

[78] Sobenin IA, Korneev NV, Romanov IV, Shutikhina IV, Kuntsevich GI, Romanenko EB, Myasoedova VA, Revin VV, Orekhov AN. The effects of garlic powder tablets in subclinical carotid atherosclerosis. Exp Clin Cardiol 2014; 20: 629–638.

[79] Libby P. Inflammation in atherosclerosis. Arterioscler Thromb Vasc Biol 2012; 32: 2045–2051.

[80] Wolf D, Stachon P, Bode C, Zirlik A. Inflammatory mechanisms in atherosclerosis. Hamostaseologie 2014; 34: 63–71.

[81] Gorchakova T, Suprun I, Sobenin I, Orekhov A. The suppression of the inflammatory cytokines expression by natural substances. Atherosclerosis 2005; 6: 66–67.

[82] Gorchakova TV, Suprun IV, Sobenin IA, Orekhov AN. Use of natural products in anticytokine therapy. Bull Exp Biol Med 2007; 143: 316–319.

[83] Gorchakova TV, Sobenin IA, Orekhov AN. The reduction of proinflammatory cytokine expression by natural components: a new approach to the prevention and treatment of atherosclerosis at the cellular level. J Clin Lipidol 2007; 1: 492.

[84] Gorchakova TV, Suprun IV, Sobenin IA, Orekhov AN. Combined anti-inflammatory and anti-atherogenic activity of natural drug Inflaminat – a perspective for long-term atherosclerosis prevention and treatment. Atherosclerosis Suppl 2007; 8: 224.

[85] Gorchakova T, Myasoedova, Sobenin I, Orekhov A. Atherosclerosis prevention with the anti-inflammatory dietary supplement Inflaminat. Atherosclerosis Suppl 2009; 10: 387.

[86] Sobenin IA, Nikitina NA, Myasoedova VA, Korennaya VV, Khalilov EG, Orekhov AN. Antiatherogenic properties of isoflavones from phytoestrogen-rich botanicals. Atherosclerosis Suppl 2003; 4: 339.

[87] Korennaya VV, Myasoedova VA, Nikitina NA, Sobenin IA, Orekhov AN. Bioflavonoid-rich botanicals reduce blood serum atherogenicity in perimenopausal women. Atherosclerosis Suppl 2006; 7: 444.

[88] Nikitina NA, Sobenin IA, Myasoedova VA, Korennaya VV, Mel'nichenko AA, Khalilov EM, Orekhov AN. Antiatherogenic effect of grape flavonoids in an *ex vivo* model. Bull Exp Biol Med. 2006; 141: 712–715.

[89] Sobenin IA, Myasoedova VA, Orekhov AN. Antiatherogenic action of isoflavonoid-rich botanicals: an implementation for atherosclerosis prevention in postmenopausal women. J Clin Lipidol 2007; 491.

[90] Myasoedova VA, Sobenin IA. Background, rationale and design of clinical study of the effect of isoflavonoid-rich botanicals on natural history of atherosclerosis in women. Atherosclerosis Suppl 2008; 9: 171.

[91] Sobenin I, Myasoedova V, Orekhov A. Atherosclerosis prevention in postmenopausal women with the isoflavonoid-rich dietary supplement Karinat. J Clin Lipidol 2008; 2: S26–27.

Chapter 3

Influence of Atorvastatin on Plasma Atherogenic Biomarkers

Marek Kucera, Stanislav Oravec and Ludovit Gaspar

Additional information is available at the end of the chapter

http://dx.doi.org/10.5772/64794

Abstract

Patients (n = 40) with hypercholesterolaemia (29 females), mean age 63 years, without previous lipid lowering treatment, were treated with atorvastatin 40 mg/day for 3 months. Total cholesterol (TC), low-density lipoprotein cholesterol (LDL-C), high-density lipoprotein cholesterol (HDL-C), triglycerides (TG), LDL-C subfractions (large LDL-C and small dense LDL-C particles), apolipoprotein A1 (apo A1), apolipoprotein B (apo B), apo B/apo A1 ratio, atherogenic index of plasma (AIP), haematological parameters including mean platelet volume (MPV), and red cell distribution width (RDW) and safety parameters (renal and hepatic function) were measured before and after 12 weeks of atorvastatin treatment. Atorvastatin significantly reduced small dense LDL (sdLDL) fraction 3–7 and apo B. There was a negative correlation of AIP with buoyant LDL 1–2 ($r = -0.35$; $p < 0.05$) and positive with small dense LDL 3–7 ($r = 0.52$, $p < 0.001$). Administration of atorvastatin 40 mg/day in patients with hypercholesterolaemia caused a shift in small dense LDL subfractions to large, buoyant subfractions. AIP correlated better with small dense LDL than apo B levels. At baseline, a strong correlation between HDL-C, TG, small dense LDL-C, apo B, apo B/apo A1 and AIP with MPV was found. After 12 weeks of treatment with atorvastatin, MPV and RDW values underwent significant modification only in those patients displaying the strongest lipid-lowering effect. Values of MPV and RDW seem to reflect a pro-atherogenic lipoprotein profile mainly represented by the presence of small dense LDL-C. No serious atorvastatin adverse events were noted.

Keywords: atorvastatin, small dense LDL, atherogenic dyslipidaemia, mean platelet volume, red cell distribution width

INTECH
open science | open minds

1. Introduction

Abnormal lipid metabolism preceding overt atherosclerosis is associated with increased cardiovascular risk. In atherogenic dyslipidaemia, the lipoprotein abnormalities include increased small dense LDL particles (sdLDL), elevations of VLDL and low HDL-cholesterol usually occur together [1, 2]. Over the last two decades, it has been demonstrated that routine measurement of total cholesterol, LDL-C and HDL-C fails to distinguish all lipoprotein abnormalities associated with cardiovascular diseases [3]. There is a need to find new biomarkers for this. By contrast, the analysis of lipoprotein subfractions appears more important in assessing the risk of cardiovascular complications [4]. LDL-C remains the primary focus for cardiovascular risk assessment and evaluation of pharmacologic effectiveness, but not based on LDL targets instead on LDL lowering [5]. Yet, a large body of evidence indicates that a narrow focus on LDL-C assessment and treatment alone is not the optimal strategy for patient care [6]. Examining individual lipoprotein subpopulations/subfractions provides opportunities for risk stratification, independent of commonly determined lipid parameters [7].

2. Plasma atherogenic biomarkers

The term "lipid triad" has been introduced to describe a common form of dyslipidaemia, characterized by three lipid abnormalities: increased plasma triglyceride levels, decreased HDL-cholesterol concentrations and the presence of sdLDL particles [8]. Apolipoprotein B (apo B) is the major protein of all lipoproteins except for high-density lipoprotein. Estimation of apo B reflects the total number of sdLDL particles. It is notable that LDL particles can vary in size, cholesterol content and number, for a given concentration of LDL-C.

Haematological parameters, mainly red cell distribution width (RDW) and mean platelet volume (MPV) have gained great interest in cardiovascular research. This has been reported to be a strong and independent predictor of adverse cardiovascular outcomes in the general population [9]. In the last few years, MPV, respected an effective marker of platelet activation, has also created much interest in cardiovascular research. This stems from the fact that platelets undergo a dramatic change in shape from quiescent discs to swollen spheres, with an increased MPV, during the activation process. It is well-known that large platelets are more adhesive and prone to aggregate than smaller ones [10], and elevated MPV values have been reported in cardiovascular diseases [11]. "Another haematological parameter which seems to play a role is RDW, a measure of the variability of red cell size. RDW has been reported to be a strong and independent predictor of adverse cardiovascular outcomes in the general population" [12].

The aim of our study was to compare different methods in the evaluation of atherogenicity, including that of the detailed lipid profile.

3. Analytic system

Various methods have been developed such as gradient gel electrophoresis, ultracentrifugation, magnetic resonance spectroscopy, endothelial models for testing lipoprotein cytotoxicity to identify atherogenic lipoproteins [13], but because of technical and financial limitations, long-term analyses and high operating costs, the previously mentioned methods were used primarily in basic research. Electrophoresis of plasma lipoproteins on the polyacrylamide gel (PAG) Lipoprint LDL system is a new method, which has become a milestone in routine laboratory analysis and in diagnosing disorders of lipoproteins, for the identification and quantitative evaluation of lipoprotein subfractions, i.e., the atherogenic and non-atherogenic lipoproteins [14]. The benefits of Lipoprint LDL method are in unique identification of an atherogenic and non-atherogenic lipoprotein spectrum in case of hyperlipoproteinaemia with the possibility of a better assessment of the adequacy of lipid-lowering interventions. Another important aspect is to identify the atherogenic lipoprotein profile in patients with normolipidaemia after lipid-lowering therapy [15].

4. Cholesterol lowering, atherogenic biomarker alteration and therapy

Clinical trials with statins have demonstrated significant reductions in cardiovascular events. Although the benefit of statin therapy has generally been ascribed to reduction in LDL-C, other atherogenic classes of lipoproteins may be beneficially affected by statin therapy [16]. The beneficial effects of atorvastatin treatment have been known for a long time although, the effect of atorvastatin on other classes of atherogenic lipoproteins has not been well studied. Previous studies, which were performed in limited trials of patients with atorvastatin 10 and 20 mg, resulted in a shift from small to large atherogenic particles of low-density lipoprotein (LDL) [17, 18]. We know that atorvastatin can improve lipoprotein metabolism, however, the medication affects different aspects of lipoprotein metabolism.

Lipid lowering treatment changes the sizes and concentrations of subtype lipoproteins and the values of some haematological parameters. There are more another favourable effects of statins in regulation of coagulation, inflammation and vascular function instead reducing LDL-C [19, 20]. Therefore, the influence of atorvastatin in decreasing cardiovascular risk could be through reduction of MPV levels. The antiplatelet and anti-inflammatory effect of atorvastatin could play a role in decreasing cardiovascular risk by reduction of MPV levels [21]. Patients with low HDL-C have significantly higher levels of MPV [22]. Likewise, the negative association has been revealed between increased RDW and low HDL-C values evaluated in large outpatient trials [23]. However, there are little data evaluating the association between MPV, RDW and low-density lipoproteins values.

A further aim of the present survey was to identify the relationship between low-density lipoprotein subfractions and haematologic parameters. The point of interest was to examine whether MPV and RDW have predictive potential for plasma levels and composition of pro- or anti-atherogenic lipoproteins. A cohort of 40 patients with hypercholesterolaemia (29 females, mean age 62.9 ± 9 years), without previous hypolipidaemic treatment were enrolled. The patients were treated with atorvastatin 40 mg/day for 12 weeks. There was documented hypercholesterolaemia in 21 patients, combined with hyperlipoproteinaemia in 19 of those.

4.1. Study design

All participants signed informed content and went through a screening protocol which included evaluation of their medical history, physical examination and testing for standard haematologic and biochemical analysis. Exclusion criteria were a history of diabetes mellitus, glomerular filtration rate less than 60 ml/min (estimated glomerular filtration rate using MDRD equation [GFR] < 60 ml/min) and liver abnormalities (abnormal AST, ALT, history of hepatopathy or cirrhosis), history of acute myocardial infarction or stroke, hypothyroidism or hyperthyroidism (abnormal TSH), cancer, history of pancreatitis, alcohol or drug abuse, systemic connective tissue diseases, history of anaemia, red blood cell transfusion, supplementation of iron, folate or stimulation of erythropoiesis. Patients were eligible to take part in the study if they met the criteria of the National Cholesterol Education Program-Adult Treatment Panel 3 (NCEP-ATP3) [24]. None of the patients involved in the study were treated with a statin before, even though some already had a diagnosis of hypertension or ischaemic heart disease. Physical and laboratory examinations were carried out after first, second and third month of treatment. The study was approved by the local ethics committee of the University Hospital in Bratislava and was conducted in accordance with the Declaration of Helsinki.

4.2. Measurements

Blood samples were drawn from the cubital vein in the morning after 12 h fasting period. Monitoring included laboratory screening (liver and renal function, glucose, electrolytes, thyroid stimulating hormone), identification of plasma atherogenity—apolipoprotein B, apolipoprotein A1, ratio apo B/apo A1 by immunoturbidimetric method (Roche, Germany) and atherogenic index of plasma (AIP) using the formula log (triglycerides [TG]/high-density lipoprotein cholesterol [HDL-C]).

The lipoprotein subpopulations—VLDL (very low-density lipoprotein), IDL (intermediate density lipoprotein): IDL1, IDL2, IDL3 (the PAG method separates the intermediate-density lipoprotein particles into three midbands MID-C, MID-B and MID-A on figures), LDL 1 to LDL 7 and HDL (high-density lipoprotein) were determined by the linear electrophoresis in polyacrylamide gel (Quantimetrix Lipoprint LDL System and Quantimetrix, California, USA). The type of lipoprotein spectrum was determined as non-atherogenic profile versus atherogenic profile. LDL 1 and LDL 2 were classified as large particles (non-atherogenic) and LDL 3 to 7 as sdLDL particles (atherogenic).

Haematological variables (including MPV, RDW) before and after treatment were measured by cell analysers (Sysmex Haematology Analyzer XP-2000i, Japan). The normal range of MPV (fl) and RDW (%) in our laboratory was 7.8–11 and 10.0–15.2, respectively. The blood samples

http://dx.doi.org/10.5772/64794

were collected in tripotassium EDTA tubes and time delay between sampling and data analysis was strictly controlled to be less than 2 h.

4.3. Statistical analysis

GraphPad Prism 5 software for Windows was used. The D'Agostino Pearson test and Kolmogorov-Smirnov test were used to verify the normal distribution of parameters in the cohort. Continuous variables were expressed as mean ± SD or median and interquartile range. We used Spearman's and Pearson's correlation analyses. For the 40 patients who were studied before and after 3 months of atorvastatin treatment, unpaired *t* tests were performed to compare apo A1, apo B, AIP and serum lipoproteins at baseline versus after 3 months of treatment. The effect of 12 weeks treatment with atorvastatin on lipid and haematological parameters was evaluated by using paired *t* test and Wilcoxon matched-pairs signed rank test. A two-tailed probability level <0.05 was considered significant.

4.4. Results

Patients in the study were diagnosed with dyslipoproteinaemia, in which 52.5% patients (n = 21) was found isolated hypercholesterolaemia and the other patients (47.5%, n = 19) combined with hyperlipidaemia. Isolated hypertriglyceridaemia was not detected. The baseline characteristics of the participants are presented in **Table 1**. When structuring groups of patients according to atherogenic and non-atherogenic lipoprotein profiles, hypercholesterolaemia without the presence of sdLDL was found in 29 subjects (72.5%), atherogenic sdLDL in 11 persons (27.5%), whereas 42% of patients with combined hyperlipaemia (n = 8) and only 14% of patients with isolated hypercholesterolaemia (n = 3) had atherogenic lipoprotein profile phenotype. We also observed 35% (n = 14) of individuals with hyperlipoproteinaemia LDL 1, 2 with non-atherogenic lipoprotein profile phenotype.

	Men		**Women**	
Number *n* (%)	11 (27.5%)		29 (72.5%)	
	Min–max	Mean ± SD	Min–max	Mean ± SD
Age (years)	42–72	60 ± 9.0	47–85	63.6 ± 9.1
BMI (kg/m²)	23.2–33.7	28.6 ± 3.1	20.8–39.1	26.7 ± 4.7
Waist (cm)	78–108	94.6 ± 12.0	74.0–113.0	87.2 ± 10.2
Smokers, *n* (%)	4 (36.4%)		4 (13.8%)	
CAD, *n* (%)	2 (18.2%)		4 (13.8%)	
Arterial hypertension, *n* (%)	8 (72.5%)		22 (75.9%)	
Obesity, *n* (%)	3 (27.3%)		6 (20.7%)	

BMI, body mass index; CAD, coronary artery disease; SD, standard deviation.

Table 1. Baseline characteristics of patients included in the study.

	AIP	apo B	apo A1	apo B/apo A1
LDL 1–2	−0.35	0.54	0.13	0.358
	$p < 0.05$	$p < 0.001$	NS	$p < 0.05$
sdLDL 3–7	0.52	0.64	−0.23	0.62
	$p < 0.001$	$p < 0.001$	NS	$p < 0.001$
HDL	−0.75	−0.43	0.58	−0.60
	$p - 0.001$	$p < 0.05$	$p < 0.001$	$p < 0.001$
IDL 1–3	0.14	0.19	−0.19	0.18
	NS	$p < 0.05$	NS	NS

AIP, atherogenic index of plasma; apo, apolipoprotein; LDL, low-density lipoprotein; sdLDL, small dense low-density lipoproteins; HDL, high-density lipoprotein; IDL, intermediate density lipoprotein; NS, not significant.

Table 2. Correlation between subpopulations and AIP, apo B, apo A1 and apo B/apo A1.

	Before treatment	After treatment	*p*
TC (mmol/l)	6.7 ± 1.0	4.6 ± 1.3	<0.001
TG (mmol/l)	1.8 ± 0.9	1.5 ± 1.0	<0.05
LDL-C (mmol/l)	4.3 ± 1.0	2.6 ± 0.9	<0.001
HDL-C (mmol/l)	1.4 ± 0.4	1.2 ± 0.3	<0.001
apo A1 (g/l)	1.68 ± 0.26	1.63 ± 0.25	NS
apo B (g/l)	1.00 ± 0.25	0.74 ± 0.22	<0.001
apo B/apo A1	0.59 ± 0.20	0.45 ± 0.16	<0.001
AIP	0.03 ± 0.30	0.03 ± 0.31	NS
Fasting glucose (mmol/l)	5.69 ± 1.31	5.69 ± 1.53	NS
hsCRP (mg/l)	3.20 ± 3.58	2.24 ± 2.65	<0.05
BMI (kg/m^2)	27.2 ± 4.3	26.9 ± 4.3	<0.05
Waist (cm)	89.2 ± 11.1	88.7 ± 11.1	NS
SBP (mmHg)	131.2 ± 12.4	126.6 ± 9.4	<0.05
DBP (mmHg)	76.4 ± 8.8	72.9 ± 9.3	<0.05
VLDL (mmol/l)	0.95 ± 0.36	0.67 ± 0.32	<0.001
IDL 1–3 (mmol/l)	1.63 ± 0.38	1.16 ± 0.33	<0.001
LDL 1–2 (mmol/l)	2.50 ± 0.76	1.55 ± 0.65	<0.001
sdLDL 3–7 (mmol/l)	0.22 ± 0.32	0.09 ± 0.16	<0.001

TC, total cholesterol; TG, triglycerides; LDL, low-density lipoprotein; sdLDL, small dense low-density lipoproteins; HDL, high-density lipoprotein; apo A1, apolipoprotein A1; apo B, apolipoprotein B; AIP, atherogenic index of plasma; SBP, systolic blood pressure; DBP, diastolic blood pressure; BMI, body mass index; hsCRP, highly sensitivity C-reactive protein; VLDL, very low-density lipoprotein; IDL, intermediate density lipoprotein.

Table 3. Effect of atorvastatin on lipids, apolipoproteins, fasting glucose, hsCRP, AIP and other parameters.

We observed a positive correlation between apo B and sdLDL 3–7 ($r = 0.64$, $p < 0.001$), and with LDL 1–2 ($r = 0.54$, $p < 0.001$). AIP showed a negative correlation with LDL 1–2 ($r = -0.35$, $p < 0.05$) and was positively correlated with sdLDL 3–7 ($r = 0.52$, $p < 0.001$; **Table 2**). There was a non-significant change of the atherogenic index of plasma (0.03 ± 0.30 versus 0.03 ± 0.31, $p = 0.142$), significant decrease in high-sensitivity C-reactive protein (hsCRP) (3.20 ± 3.58 versus 2.24 ± 2.65 mg/l, $p < 0.05$) and body mass index (BMI) (27.2 ± 4.3 versus 26.9 ± 4.3 kg/m^2, $p < 0.05$; **Table 3**).

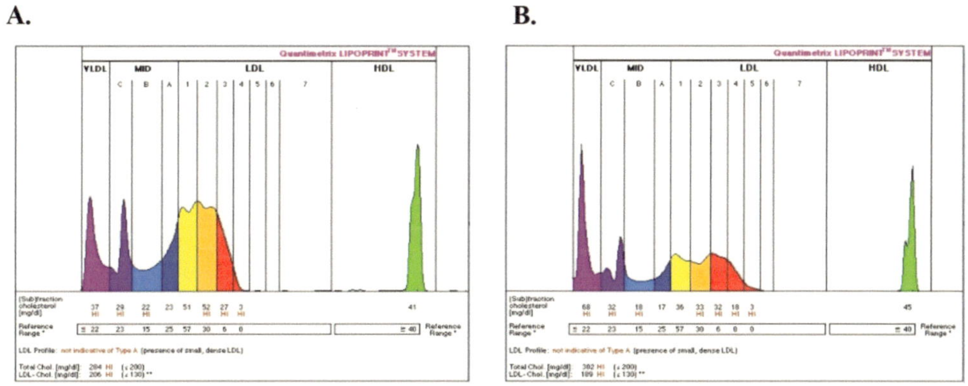

Figure 1. Distribution of lipoproteins using polyacrylamide gel method before (A) and after (B) treatment with atorvastatin 40 mg. Atherogenic lipoproteins are present despite treatment (MID-C is IDL-1, MID-B is IDL-2 and MID-A is IDL-3).

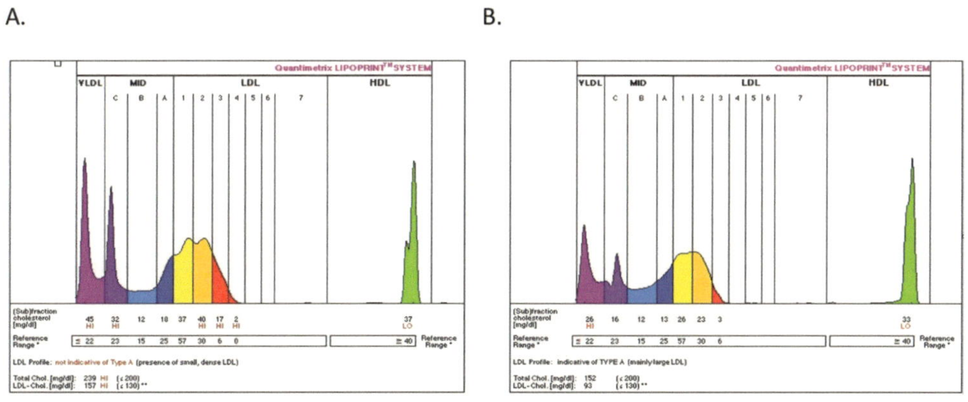

Figure 2. Reduction of lipoprotein subpopulations after treatment (B) with atorvastatin 40 mg compared with baseline lipid lipoprotein profile (A). There is fall in the atherogenic LDL 3–7 fraction after treatment (MID-C is IDL-1, MID-B is IDL-2 and MID-A is IDL-3).

Despite lipid-lowering therapy and normal values of lipids, the Lipoprint LDL method revealed presence of sdLDL (**Figure 1**). Atorvastatin significantly reduced the presence of sdLDL 3–7 (0.22 ± 0.37 versus 0.09 ± 0.16 mmol/l, $p < 0.001$), as well as other subpopulations of lipoproteins (LDL 1–2, VLDL, IDL 1–3; **Figure 2**). Atorvastatin 40 mg had little effect on the initial subfractions LDL 1 and LDL 2 (**Figure 3**). The proportion of buoyant and sdLDL at baseline was 11.36 mmol/l ($p < 0.001$) and after treatment 17.22 mmol/l ($p < 0.001$).

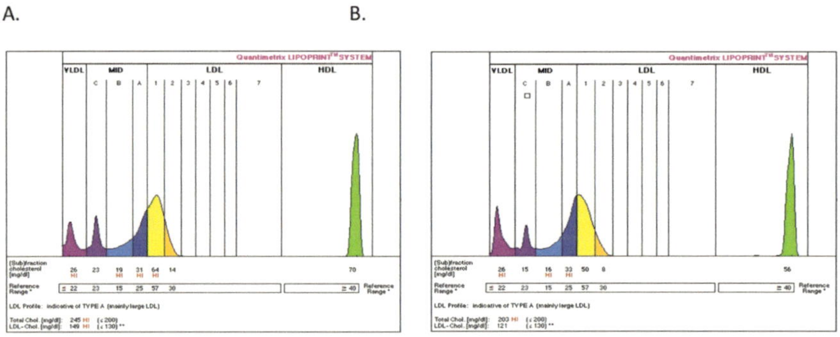

Figure 3. Effect of atorvastatin 40 mg on hyperbetalipoproteinaemia before (A) and after treatment (B). There were no changes in lipoprotein profile after treatment (MID-C is IDL-1, MID-B is IDL-2 and MID-A is IDL-3).

Haematological parameters	Before treatment Mean ± SD/Median [IQR]	After treatment Mean ± SD/Median [IQR]	P
RBC (10^{12}/l)	4.16 [3.9–4.7]	4.12 [3.9—4.69]	NS
Haemoglobin (g/l)	143.0 [139.0–148.8]	143.0 [137.3–147.8]	NS
MCV (fl)	90.45 [89.03–92.1]	90.0 [88.93–91.52]	NS
RDW (%)	12.75 [11.0–15.5]	12.4 [10.85–15.35]	NS
Platelet (10^9/l)	288.0 [217.0–300.5]	288.0 [256.5–309.8]	<0.05
MPV (fl)	8.65 [8.03–10.68]	8.80 [8.33–9.63]	NS
WBC (10^9/l)	6.42 [5.91–7.4]	6.6 [6.0–7.34]	NS

RBC, red blood cell count; MCV, mean cell volume; RDW, red cell distribution width; MPV, medium platelet volume; WBC, white blood cell count; IQR, interquartile range; *r*, correlation index.
$p < 0.05$ was significant; NS, non-significant.

Table 4. Comparison of haematological parameters before and after atorvastatin treatment.

In all subjects, atorvastatin treatment was administered as either primary or secondary prevention. By contrast, no significant changes of the selected haematological parameters were observed after statin intervention, except for platelet count (**Table 4**). However, when applying the correlation analysis, a strong association between the haematological parameters and plasma lipids was evident at baseline and after 12 weeks of statin therapy (**Tables 5** and **6**). In particular, in the subgroup of patients ($n = 25$) experiencing the greatest lipid-lowering effect, as determined by the reduction of sdLDL-C, a statistically significant decline of MPV ($p = 0.006$) was observed. A positive association between the levels of sdLDL-C and MPV in this cohort was clearly evident at baseline ($r = 0.83$, $p < 0.001$) and after therapy ($r = 0.7$, $p < 0.001$; **Table 7**). In addition, haemoglobin and platelet count appeared modified following a course of statin treatment ($p = 0.003$, $p = 0.03$, respectively) in this subgroup of patient. Atorvastatin was well-tolerated during the study. No serious adverse events were noted.

Baseline	MPV	RDW	After treatment	MPV	RDW
Total cholesterol	$r = 0.04$	$r = 0.10$	**Total cholesterol**	$r = -0.03$	$r = 0.05$
	NS	NS		NS	NS
LDL-C	$r = 0.07$	$r = 0.08$	**LDL-C**	$r = -0.19$	$r = 0.07$
	NS	NS		NS	NS
HDL-C	$r = -0.55$	$r = -0.49$	**HDL-C**	$r = -0.37$	$r = -0.39$
	$p < 0.001$	$p < 0.001$		$p < 0.05$	$p < 0.05$
TG	$r = 0.57$	$r = 0.62$	**TG**	$r = 0.31$	$r = 0.39$
	$p < 0.001$	$p < 0.001$		$p < 0.05$	$p < 0.05$

LDL-C, low-density lipoprotein; HDL-C, high-density lipoprotein; TG, triglycerides; MPV, medium platelet volume; RDW, red cell distribution width; *r*, correlation index; NS, non-significant.
$p < 0.05$ was significant.

Table 5. Correlation between values of plasma lipids and haematological parameters at baseline and after treatment.

Baseline	MPV	RDW	After treatment	MPV	RDW
LDL 1–2	$r = -0.05$	$r = -0.21$	**LDL 1–2**	$r = 0.01$	$r = 0.12$
	NS	NS		NS	NS
sdLDL 3–7	$r = 0.73$	$r = 0.67$	**sdLDL 3–7**	$r = 0.54$	$r = 0.56$
	$p < 0.001$	$p < 0.001$		$p < 0.001$	$p < 0.001$
IDL 1–3	$r = -0.05$	$r = 0.04$	**IDL 1–3**	$r = -0.21$	$r = 0.1$
	NS	NS		NS	NS
apo_B	$r = 0.41$	$r = 0.41$	**apo B**	$r = -0.03$	$r = 0.26$
	$p < 0.05$	$p < 0.05$		NS	NS
apo_A1	$r = -0.36$	$r = -0.24$	**apo_A1**	$r = -0.19$	$r = -0.26$
	$p < 0.05$	NS		NS	NS
apo B/apo A1	$r = 0.52$	$r = 0.43$	**apo B/apo_A1**	$r = 0.03$	$r = 0.39$
	$p < 0.001$	$p < 0.05$		NS	$p < 0.05$
AIP	$r = 0.61$	$r = 0.65$	**AIP**	$r = 0.36$	$r = 0.41$
	p < 0.001	$p < 0.001$		$p < 0.05$	$p < 0.05$

LDL, low-density lipoprotein; sdLDL, small dense low-density lipoproteins; IDL, intermedium density lipoprotein; apo_B, apolipoprotein B; apo_A1, apolipoprotein A1; AIP, atherogenic index of plasma; MPV, medium platelet volume; RDW, red cell distribution width; *r*, correlation index; NS, non-significant.
$p < 0.05$ was significant.

Table 6. Correlation between lipoproteins, apolipoproteins, AIP and haematological parameters at baseline and after treatment.

Haematological parameters in the subgroup (n n == 25)	Before treatment Mean ± SD/Median [IOR]	After treatment Mean ± SD/Median [IOR]	p
RBC (10^{12}/l)	4.46 ± 0.46	4.44 ± 0.46	NS
Haemoglobin (g/l)	145.8 ± 5.61	144.9 ± 5.81	$p < 0.05$
MCV (fl)	90.8 ± 2.15	90.21 ± 1.74	NS
RDW (%)	13.30 [12.2–15.85]	13.0 [11.5–15.8]	NS
Platelet (10^9/l)	287.0 [194.0–298.0]	287.0 [209.0–306.0]	$p < 0.05$
MPV (fl)	9.9 [8.4–10.9]	8.9 [8.45–9.85]	$p < 0.05$
WBC (10^9/l)	6.34 [5.98–6.95]	6.6 [5.95–6.8]	NS

RBC, red blood cell count; MCV, mean cell volume; RDW, red cell distribution width; MPV, medium platelet volume; WBC, white blood cell count; IQR, interquartile range; *r*, correlation index; NS, non-significant.
$p < 0.05$ was significant.

Table 7. Comparison of haematological parameters before and after atorvastatin treatment.

4.5. Discussion

Over last decade, evidence from clinic trials indicates that broad-based treatment of dyslipidaemia can improve the event-free survival rate in people who already have clinical cardiovascular diseases [25]. However, assessment of atherogenesis requires the quantification small dense lipoproteins both in patients with hyperlipoproteinaemia and normolipaemia. The decrease in HDL-C level we observed requires further study. It also seems necessary to focus on the changes of HDL subpopulations during lipid-lowering therapy [26]. A substantial residual cardiovascular risk persists, despite best treatment efforts [27–29]. We observed a 35% occurrence of hyperlipoproteinaemia LDL 1 and LDL 2 with non-atherogenic lipoprotein profile phenotype A in our patients. LDL 1 and LDL 2 are less atherogenic or not atherogenic at all and are responsible for the transport of cholesterol [30]. The presence of LDL 1 and LDL 2 in serum in the optimal concentration is essential for the normal function of endocrine organs with steroidogenesis, but also for the formation of bile acids, vitamin D3, enzymes of lipid metabolism and cell renewal of membrane structures. Within cells, cholesterol is important precursor molecule for several biochemical pathways. There is necessary for their physiological processes in the body [31]. It would be desirable for future studies to directly explain this non-atherogenic hyperbetalipoproteinaemia LDL1,2 in hypercholesterolaemic subjects with cardiometabolic diseases.

"Atherogenic normolipidaemia" after statin therapy is crucial, as this profile may increase cardiovascular risk. However, the usefulness of searching for atherogenic lipoproteins in these patients requires further research. "Atherogenic normolipaemia" was not present in our subjects, because we chose the patients for atorvastatin therapy according to the recommendations for the treatment of dyslipoproteinaemia [32, 33]. However, a breakthrough in the stage of subclinical atherosclerosis may not occur unless we are able to clearly quantify atherogenic lipoproteins both in patients with hyperlipoproteinaemia and normolipaemia.

In our study, a correlation between apo B and lipoproteins was determined. Apo B was raised not only in the presence of sdLDL 3–7 but also in the case of large LDL 1–2 particles. The only protein component of LDL is a single molecule of apo B-100 per particle [34]. Apolipoprotein B therefore cannot provide direct information about the density and size of particles in patients in whom excess of sdLDL particles can be expected [33]. This is not common practice. Therefore, the number of LDL particles could be more important in terms of risk than particle size in itself as a better option for diagnosis of atherogenic particles. If further studies this option confirmed, it seems that the easiest marker of atherogenicity could be the AIP [35]. Our results show a significant change in LDL particle size (from larger and cholesterol-rich to smaller and cholesterol-poor) after atorvastatin treatment. We wanted to point out the persistence of "atherogenic normolipaemia" and hypercholesterolaemia in some patients irrespective of statin therapy. Therefore, qualitative determination of lipoproteins after lipid-lowering therapy was the aim of the study [36].

A lot of evidence support that statins have pleiotropic effects beyond their cholesterol-lowering activity [37, 38]. For instance, statins modulate platelet function via direct interactions with platelet membranes [39] or regulation of platelet signalling pathways [40]. Increased platelets activity is crucial in pathophysiology of atherothrombosis. Recent reports showed that statins involve the inhibition of calcium-dependent phospholipase A2 (cPLA2) [41], the activation of nitric oxide synthase [42], and the accumulation of cAMP [43] in the anti-aggregation. Treatment with atorvastatin or simvastatin also causes down-regulation of the expression of CD36 and LOX-1, the reduction of platelet-associated oxidized LDL level [44] and thromboxane A2 and B2 formation [39], and the inhibition of NADPH oxidase (Nox2) [45].

Although MPV is parameter of platelet size, it is considered as a marker of platelet reactivity [46]. Sivri et al. reported that MPV significantly decreased after statin treatment for the irrespective of cholesterol levels [47]. Recent trial indicates the effect of rosuvastatin on MPV level although the changes were not correlated with the plasma lipids which may reflect significant anti-platelet activation properties [48]. Similarly to previous study, the work with atorvastatin has revealed possible relation of statin treatment and MPV [21]. We found that there were no effect of 12 weeks atorvastatin therapy on MPV and RDW, but in the subgroup of patients (n = 25) with the decrease in sdLDL-C after statin treatment, we have observed significant reduction in MPV (**Table 7**).

The question of how we could decrease MPV has already been raised [49]. It has been revealed that the lipid-lowering effect of statin therapy is not involved in inhibition of thrombus formation in hypercholesterolaemic subjects. Previous finding suggests that other lipid-independent effects of statins may contribute to their anti-aggregatory activity [50]. A limitation of MPV, as a prognostic marker, is uncertain up-to-date as the relationship between platelet size and cardiovascular risk is causative or is only a secondary effect.

The RDW is a measurement of cell size distribution and is commonly requested test used for variety of purposes, for instance to distinguish aneamias [51]. Recent work has revealed a strong correlation between elevated RDW and the occurrence of fatal and nonfatal cardiovascular events [52]. Complete blood count risk score including RDW was strongly associated with all-cause mortality in the JUPITER study in primary populations initially free from cardiovascular disease [53]. Recently, Lippi et al. [23] reported a significant association of increased RDW and low HDL-C, as well as relation with high TG and high AIP involving 4874 unselected outpatients. An interventional study of 79 patients treated with atorvastatin (10–80 mg) for 24-week period has not shown significant RDW changes [21]. It remains still unknown which physiological process leads to previous outcomes, although inflammation has been reported as possible cause [54]. Therefore, there might be a new and unpredictable scenario in the clinical usefulness of RDW.

It has been suggested that cardiovascular risk may be more closely related to atherogenic lipoprotein profile mostly represented by presence of sdLDL-C particles [55]. To our knowledge, the present study was the first to analyse MPV and RDW in relation to concentration of lipoprotein subfractions, especially with sdLDL-C. The main finding was that MPV and RDW correlated with sdLDL-C and in subgroup of sdLDL-C lowering effect after treatment, indeed, there was significant decrease in MPV value (**Table 6**). This may indicate that subjects with more a pronounced lipid-lowering effect after statin treatment may benefit also from effects beyond this well-known action. We have also observed that platelet count and haemoglobin value have changed significantly after statin therapy in this subgroup. However, this finding appears not to be clinically important.

The current study results suggest that MPV and RDW can play an important role not only in hypercholesterolaemia but also interfering with atherogenic small dense lipoproteins. Haematological parameters can be easily analysed at low cost and indices be new biomarkers for atherosclerosis. The potential problems that may concern is that various studies revealed the significance of MPV or RDW about the presence of various diseases and confounding factors (obesity, smoking, arterial hypertension, inflammation diseases, pulmonary embolism, etc.). Its clinical significance, however, remains largely difficult. There is still a need for further prospective, multicentre studies with a large sample size to fully clarify the issue.

Acknowledgements

This work was supported by a grant from the European Regional Development Fund—Project FNUSA-ICRC (No. CZ.1.05/1.1.00/02.0123). We would like to acknowledge the excellent technical assistance of all participants from 2nd Department of Internal Medicine, Faculty of Medicine, Comenius University, Bratislava, Slovak Republic.

Conflict of interest and funding

The authors declare no conflict of interest and have not received any funding or benefits from industry or any for profit organization for this work.

Author details

Marek Kucera*, Stanislav Oravec and Ludovit Gaspar

*Address all correspondence to: marekucera@gmail.com

2nd Department of Internal Medicine, Comenius University in Bratislava, Slovak Republic

References

[1] Musunuru K. Atherogenic dyslipidemia: cardiovascular risk and dietary intervention. Lipids. 2010; 45: 907–14.

[2] Gang H, Qing Q, Tuomilehto J, et al. Prevalence of the metabolic syndrome and its relation to all-cause and cardiovascular mortality in nondiabetic European men and women. Arch Intern Med. 2004; 164(10): 1066–76.

[3] Ridker PM, Rifai N, Cook NR, Bradwin G, Buring JE. Non-HDL cholesterol, apolipoproteins A-I and B100, standard lipid measures, lipid ratios, and CRP as risk factors for cardiovascular disease in women. JAMA. 2005; 20: 326–33.

[4] Oravec S, Dukat A, Gavornik P, et al. Atherogenic versus non-atherogenic lipoprotein profiles in healthy individuals. is there a need to change our approach to diagnosing dyslipidemia? Curr Med Chem. 2014; 21(25): 2892–901.

[5] Gulati M, Merz CN. New cholesterol guidelines and primary prevention in women. Trends Cardiovasc Med. 2015; 25(2): 84–94.

[6] Oravec S, Gruber K, Dukat A, et al. The assessment of the atherogenic lipoprotein profile in cardiovascular diseases by lipoprint system analysis. In: Kostner G, Chennamesetty I, editors. Biochemistry, Genetics and Molecular Biology "Lipoproteins—From Bench to Bedside". Croatia: InTech; 2015. p. 87–111.

[7] Oravec S, Gruber K, Dostal E. Hyper-betalipoproteinemia LDL 1,2: a newly identified nonatherogenic hypercholesterolemia in a group of hypercholesterolemic subjects. Neuro Endocrinol Lett. 2011; 32(3): 322–7.

[8] Rizzo M, Berneis K. Lipid triad or atherogenic lipoprotein phenotype: a role in cardiovascular prevention? J Atheroscler Thromb. 2005; 12(5): 237–9.

[9] Gijsberts CM, den Ruijter HM, de Kleijn DP, et al. Hematological parameters improve prediction of mortality and secondary adverse events in coronary angiography patients: a longitudinal cohort study. Medicine (Baltimore). 2015; 94(45):1–10.

[10] Martin JF, Trowbridge EA, Salmon G, Plumb J. The biological significance of platelet volume: its relationship to bleeding time, thromboxane B2 production and megakaryocyte nuclear DNA concentration. Thromb Res. 1983; 32: 443–60.

[11] Pizzulli L, Yang A, Martin JF, Luderttz B. Changes in platelet size and count in unstable angina compared to stable angina or non-cardiac chest pain. Eur Heart J. 1998; 19: 80–4.

[12] Perlstein TS, Weuve J, Pfeffer MA, Beckman JA. Red blood cell distribution width and mortality risk in a community-based prospective cohort. Arch Intern Med. 2009; 169: 588–94.

[13] Hirany SV, Othman Y, Kutscher P, et al. Comparison of low-density lipoprotein size by polyacrylamide tube gel electrophoresis and polyacrylamide gradient gel electrophoresis. Am J Clin Pathol. 2003; 119: 439–45.

[14] Oravec S. Identifikácia subpopulácií LDL triedy - Aktuálny prínos v diagnostike porúch metabolizmu lipoproteínov a ochorení kardiovaskulárneho systému (Identification of LDL subfractions—a contribution in the diagnostics of lipoprotein metabolism diseases and cardiovascular diseases). Med Milit Slov. 2006; 8: 32–4.

[15] Hoefner MD, Hodel DS, O'Brien FJ, et al. Development of a rapid quantitative method for LDL subfractionation with use of the Quantimetrix Lipoprint LDL system. Clin Chem. 2001; 47(2): 266–74.

[16] Maron DJ, Fazio S, Linton MF. Current perspectives on statins. Circulation. 2000; 101: 207–13.

[17] Sasaki S, Kuwahara N, Kunitomo K, et al. Effects of atorvastatin on oxidized low – density lipoprotein, low density lipoprotein subfraction distribution, and remnant lipoprotein in patients with mixed hyperlipoproteinemia. Am J Cardiol. 2002; 89(4): 386–9.

[18] Pontrelli L, Parris W, Adeli K, et al. Atorvastatin treatment beneficially alters the lipoprotein profile and increases low density lipoprotein particle diameter in patients with combined dyslipidemia and impaired fasting glucose in type 2 diabetes. Metabolism. 2002; 51(3): 334–42.

[19] Bickel C, Rupprecht HJ, Blankenberg S, Spinola-Klein C, Rippin G, Hafner G, Lotz J, Prellwitz W, Meyer J, AtheroGene Group. Influence of HMGCoA reductase inhibitors on markers of coagulation, systemic inflammation and soluble cell adhesion. Int J Cardol. 2002; 82: 25–31.

[20] Undas A, Brummel-Ziedins KE, Potaczek DP, Stobierska-Dzierzek B, Bryniarski L, Szczeklik A, Mann KG. Atorvastatin and quinapril inhibit blood coagulation in patients with coronary artery disease following 28 days of therapy. J Thromb Haemost. 2006; 11: 2397–404.

[21] Akin F, Ayca B, Köse N et al. Effect of atorvastatin on haematologic parameters in patients with hypercholesterolemia. Angiology. 2013; 64: 621–5.

[22] Varol E, Aksoy F, Bas HA, et al. Mean platelet volume is elevated in patients with low high-density lipoprotein cholesterol. Angiology. 2014; 65(8): 733–6.

[23] Lippi G, Sanchis-Gomar F, Danese E, Montagnana M. Association of red blood cell distribution width with plasma lipids in a general population of unselected outpatients. Kardiol Pol. 2013; 71: 931–6.

[24] American College of Cardiology/American Heart Association Task Force on Practice Guidelines. 2013 ACC/AHA guideline on the treatment of blood cholesterol to reduce atherosclerotic cardiovascular risk in adults. Am Coll Cardiol. 2014; 63: 2889–934.

[25] Banach M, Nikfar S, Rahimi R, et al.; Lipid and Blood Pressure Meta-Analysis Collaboration Group. The effects of statins on blood pressure in normotensive or hypertensive subjects—a meta-analysis of randomized controlled trials. Int J Cardiol. 2013; 168(3): 2816–24.

[26] Otocka-Kmiecik A, Mikhailidis DP, Nicholls SJ, Davidson M, Rysz J, Banach M. Dysfunctional HDL: a novel important diagnostic and therapeutic target in cardiovascular disease? Prog Lipid Res. 2012; 51(4): 314–24.

[27] Rizzo M, Barylski M, Rizvi AA, Montalto G, Mikhailidis DP, Banach M. Combined dyslipidemia: should the focus be LDL cholesterol or atherogenic dyslipidemia? Curr Pharm Des. 2013; 19(21): 3858–68.

[28] Rizzo M, Banach M, Montalto G, Mikhailidis DP. Lipid-lowering therapies and achievement of LDL-cholesterol targets. Arch Med Sci. 2012; 8(4): 598–600.

[29] Miller M, Cannon CP, Murphy SA, et al. Impact of triglyceride levels beyond low density lipoprotein cholesterol after acute coronary syndrome in the PROVE-IT TIMI 22 Trial. J Am Coll Cardiol. 2008; 51(7): 724–30.

[30] Oravec S. Plasma lipoproteins. In: Oravec S, editor. Lipoproteins in the diagnosis of internal diseases. Bratislava: VEDA; 1999. p. 31.

[31] Petrov AM, Zefirov AL. Cholesterol and lipid rafts in the biological membranes. Role in the release, reception and ion channel functions. Usp Fiziol Nauk. 2013; 44(1): 17–38.

[32] Banach M, Nikfar S, Rahimi R, et al.; Lipid and Blood Pressure Meta-Analysis Collaboration Group. The effects of statins on blood pressure in normotensive or hypertensive subjects—a meta-analysis of randomized controlled trials. Int J Cardiol. 2013; 168(3): 2816–24.

[33] Walldius G, Jungner I, Holme I, et al. High apolipoprotein B, low apolipoprotein A-1, and improvement in the prediction of fatal myocardial infarction (AMORIS study): a prospective study. Lancet. 2001; 15(9298): 2026–33.

[34] Mikhailidis DP, Elisaf M, Rizzo M, et al. "European panel on low density lipoprotein (LDL) subclasses": a statement on the pathophysiology, atherogenicity and clinical significance of LDL subclasses. Curr Vasc Pharmacol. 2011; 9(5): 533–71.

[35] Dobiášová M. Atherogenic index of plasma [log(triglycerides/HDL-cholesterol)]: theoretical and practical implications. Clin Chem. 2004; 50(7): 1113–5.

[36] Nikolic D, Katsiki N, Montalto G, Isenovic ER, Mikhailidis DP, Rizzo M. Lipoprotein subfractions in metabolic syndrome and obesity: clinical significance and therapeutic approaches. Nutrients. 2013; 5(3): 928–48.

[37] Liao JK. Effects of statins on 3-hydroxy-3-methylglutaryl coenzyme a reductase inhibition beyond low-density lipoprotein cholesterol. Am J Cardiol. 2005; 96: 24F–33F.

[38] Marzilli M. Pleiotropic effects of statins: evidence for benefits beyond LDL-cholesterol lowering. Am J Cardiovasc Drugs. 2010; 10(1): 3–9.

[39] Ma LP, Nie DN, Hsu SX, et al. Inhibition of platelet aggregation and expression of alpha granule membrane protein 140 and thromboxane B2 with pravastatin therapy for hypercholesterolemia. J Assoc Acad Minor Phys. 2002; 13(1): 23–6.

[40] Luzak B, Rywaniak J, Stanczyk L, Watala C. Pravastatin and simvastatin improves acetylsalicylic acid-mediated in vitro blood platelet inhibition. Eur J Clin Invest. 2012; 42(8): 864–72.

[41] Moscardó A, Vallés J, Latorre A, et al. Reduction of platelet cytosolic phospholipase A 2 activity by atorvastatin and simvastatin: biochemical regulatory mechanisms. Thromb Res. 2013; 131: e154–e159.

[42] Chou TC, Lin YF, Wu WC, Chu KM. Enhanced nitric oxide and cyclic GMP formation plays a role in the anti-platelet activity of simvastatin. Br J Pharmacol. 2008; 153: 1281–7.

[43] Lee YM, Chen WF, Chou DS, et al. Cyclic nucleotides and mitogen-activated protein kinases: regulation of simvastatin in platelet activation. J Biomed Sci. 2010; 17: 45.

[44] Bruni F, Pasqui AL, Pastorelli M, et al. Different effect of statins on platelet oxidized-LDL receptor (CD36 and LOX-1) expression in hypercholesterolemic subjects. Clin Appl Thromb Hemost. 2005; 11: 417–28.

[45] Pignatelli P, Carnevale R, Pastori D, et al. Immediate antioxidant and antiplatelet effect of atorvastatin via inhibition of Nox2. Circulation. 2012; 126(1): 92–103.

[46] Davi G, Patrono C. Platelet activation and atherothrombosis. N Engl J Med. 2007; 357: 2482–94.

[47] Sivri N, Tekin G, Yalta K, et al. Statins decrease mean platelet volume irrespective of cholesterol lowering effect. Kardiol Pol. 2013; 71: 1042–7.

[48] Coban E, Afacan B. The effect of rosuvastatin treatment on the mean platelet volume in patients with uncontrolled primary dyslipidemia with hypolipidemic diet treatment. Platelets. 2008; 19(2): 111–4.

[49] Yetkin E. Mean platelet volume not so far from being a routine diagnostic and prognostic measurement. Thromb Haemost. 2008; 100: 3–4.

[50] Gaddam V, Li DY, Mehta JL. Anti-thrombotic effects of atorvastatin—an effect unrelated to lipid lowering. J Cardiovasc Pharmacol Ther. 2002; 7: 247–53.

[51] Evans TC, Jehle D. The red blood cell distribution width. J Emerg Med. 1991; 9: 71–4.

[52] Anderson JL, Ronnow BS, Horne BD, et al. Usefulness of a complete blood count-derived risk score to predict incident mortality in patients with suspected cardiovascular disease. Am J Cardiol. 2007; 99: 169–74.

[53] Horne D, Anderson JL, Muhlstein JB, et al. JUPITER trial complete blood count risk score and its components, including RDW, are associated with mortality in the JUPITER trial. Eur J Prevent Cardiol. 2014; 22(4): 519–26.

[54] Tonelli M, Sacks F, Arnold M, et al. Relation between red blood cell distribution width and cardiovascular event rate in people with coronary disease. Circulation. 2008; 117(2): 163–8.

[55] Arai H, Kokubo Y, Watanabe M, et al. Small dense low-density lipoproteins cholesterol can predict incident cardiovascular disease in an urban Japanese cohort: the Suita study. J Atheroscler Thromb. 2013; 20: 195–203.

Chapter 4

Treatment of Homozygous Familial Hypercholesterolemia: Challenges and Latest Development

Min-Ji Charng

Additional information is available at the end of the chapter

http://dx.doi.org/10.5772/63949

Abstract

Familial hypercholesterolemia (FH) is an autosomal codominant genetic disorder of lipoprotein metabolism. Patients can be heterozygous (HeFH) with one mutated allele, homozygous (HoFH) with two identical mutations, or compound heterozygous with different mutations in each allele. HoFH is the more severe form of the disease and is associated with extremely elevated levels of total cholesterol and low-density lipoprotein cholesterol (LDL-C). These lipid abnormalities are associated with accelerated atherosclerosis and cardiovascular disease (CVD) and an increased risk of cardiac events and early death. The prevalence of HoFH has been estimated to be 1 in 1 million; however, this is likely an underestimation as the disease is substantially underdiagnosed and undertreated. Early diagnosis and treatment are important to reduce CVD events. Aggressive therapy with conventional agents such as statins and ezetimibe produce substantial reductions in LDL-C, but patients rarely reach target goals. Apheresis should be considered in all patients with HoFH, although LDL-C levels rapidly rebound to baseline levels. Three recently introduced novel agents (mipomersen, lomitapide, and evolocumab)—each with a unique mechanism of action—have increased therapeutic options in this difficult-to-treat population. When added to standard therapy, these agents produce significant additional LDL-C lowering and can potentially improve clinical outcomes.

Keywords: evolocumab, familial hypercholesterolemia, lomitapide, mipomersen, treatment

1. Introduction

Familial hypercholesterolemia (FH) is an autosomal codominant genetic disorder of lipoprotein metabolism, usually caused by mutations in the low-density lipoprotein (LDL) receptor (*LDLR*) gene or other genes that affect LDLR function. Patients can be heterozygous (HeFH) with one mutated allele, homozygous (HoFH) with two identical mutations, or compound heterozygous with different mutations in each allele [1]. Patients with HoFH have either a complete absence or marked impairment (i.e., 2–30% activity) in LDLR function [1]. There are a number of defects in lipid metabolism among patients with FH that include reduced LDLR-mediated catabolism of LDL, impairment of apolipoprotein B (apo B)-mediated clearance of LDL, and increased proprotein convertase subtilisin/kexin type 9 (PCSK9) levels, which mediates posttranslational destruction of LDLRs [2, 3].

Since the reduction of LDLRs in HoFH is more pronounced than that seen with HeFH, hypercholesterolemia is usually more severe in HoFH than in HeFH and is characterized by very high serum levels of total cholesterol and LDL-cholesterol (LDL-C). Levels of LDL-C are typically above 500 mg/dL and total cholesterol levels range from 650 to 1000 mg/dL when HoFH is untreated, whereas LDL-C levels are typically greater than 300 mg/dL when treated [2–5]. High-density lipoprotein cholesterol (HDL-C) is often decreased and triglyceride levels are generally normal [4].

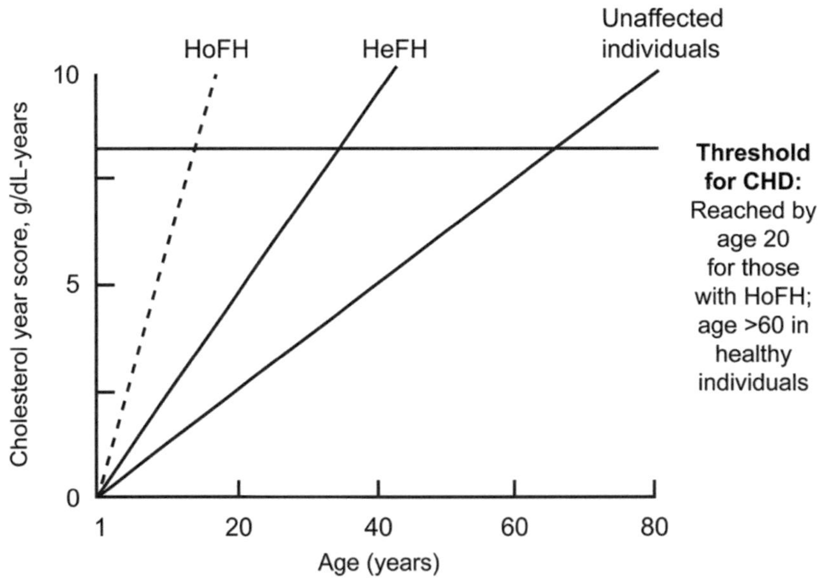

Figure 1. Cumulative LDL exposure in patients with FH [8, 9]. Modified from Horton et al. 2009 [9].

The severe lipid abnormalities associated with HoFH result in accelerated atherosclerosis, accelerated cardiovascular disease (CVD), and an increased risk of cardiac events and early death. It is estimated that CVD risk is increased by up to 20-fold in untreated patients and still elevated approximately 10-fold in patients receiving statins [5–7]. The lifelong exposure of highly elevated lipid levels means that signs/symptoms of CVD occur at an early age—typically prior to 20 years of age and as early as preteen years with the highest risk in males [5, 8]. Females develop CVD about 10 years later than males [6]. Young patients often have severe and widespread atherosclerosis in all major arterial beds, including the carotid, coronary, femoral, and iliac, and there have been instances of acute myocardial infarction and sudden death in patients as young as 4 years of age [8]. The CVD risk is related to cumulative LDL-C exposure. As seen in **Figure 1**, patients with HoFH exceed the theoretical threshold of LDL-C exposure in early childhood compared with early middle age for patients with HeFH and after age 60 years for normal healthy individuals [8, 9]. Although, as with all individuals, the risk of developing CVD is also related to the presence of other genetic or environmental risk factors, the effect of each risk factor is amplified in the setting of dramatically elevated cholesterol levels [4].

The physical signs and symptoms of HoFH are characterized by accelerated atherosclerosis and the deposition of cholesterol. Atherosclerotic manifestations include vascular endothelial damage that produces premature coronary artery disease (CAD), peripheral artery disease, and valvular disease (e.g., aortic stenosis) [4]. Deposition of cholesterol results in the development of cutaneous or tendinous xanthomas and corneal arcus [8]. Xanthomas typically occur around the eyelids and tendons of the feet, hands, and elbows [5].

HoFH is substantially underdiagnosed and undertreated [7]. For example, it is estimated that less than 1% of patients with FH are diagnosed in most countries and that only 48% of patients with FH were receiving statin therapy in one Danish study [7]. Most patients with FH are not identified because of inconsistent screening and general unawareness [6]. Indeed, the disease is often not recognized until the initial cardiovascular (CV) event [6].

2. Epidemiology

The exact prevalence rate of HoFH is unknown. Although the prevalence is historically estimated to be approximately 1 in 1 million [7], this likely underestimates true prevalence rates. More recent estimates, based on surveys of unselected general populations that found a prevalence of HeFH of 1 in ~200 or 1 in 244, suggest a prevalence of 1 in 160,000 to 1 in 300,000 for HoFH [10]. Founder mutations that reduce genetic variation can influence the prevalence in certain racial groups or geographic locations, resulting in increased prevalence in certain groups (e.g., French Canadian, the Netherlands, Lebanese, Hokuriku district of Japan, South African Afrikaners) [11–15]. National programs that include patient registries and cascade screening have been useful for identifying patients and facilitating treatments.

3. Genetics

True HoFH is caused by two identical mutations that are inherited in an autosomal dominant pattern [16]. Two mutant alleles of the *LDLR* gene (*MIM 606945*) cause the majority (85–95%)

of cases [7, 10, 17]. Mutations in this gene cause a reduction in LDLR activity and are associated with decreased clearance of LDL particles and increased LDL-C levels.

Secondary genes associated with HoFH include *APOB* (*MIM107730*), *PCSK9* (*MIM 607786*), and *LDLR-adaptor protein 1* (*LDLRAP1*; *MIM 605747*) [8, 10, 17]. In addition to "true" HoFH, patients with HoFH can have compound heterozygous mutations (different mutations in each allele of the same gene) or double heterozygous mutations (mutations in two different genes affecting LDLR function) [7, 10]. The severity of the HoFH depends on residual LDLR activity. Irrespective of the underlying genetic defect, patients with HoFH are classified as either receptor negative (i.e., <2% residual activity) or receptor defective (i.e., 2–25% residual activity) [10]. The effect on LDL-C concentrations is also related to genotype. Homozygous *LDLR*-defective mutations are generally associated with the highest LDL-C levels, followed by compound heterozygous *LDLR*-defective + *LDLR*-negative mutations, homozygous *LDLRAP1* or *LDLR*-defective mutations, homozygous *APOB* or *PCKS9* gain-of-function mutation, and double heterozygous mutation [5, 10]. Metabolic defects include impaired LDL uptake (the most common functional defect), hepatic oversecretion of apo B, decreased catabolism of triglyceride-rich lipoproteins, increased plasma levels of lipoprotein(a) (Lp(a)), and low levels of HDL-C [10].

4. Diagnosis

Since CV risk is related to the cumulative exposure to elevated lipids, early diagnosis is important for earlier treatment of HoFH to reduce CV risk. Although genetic testing can confirm FH, it is not well defined since genetic confirmation can be difficult to verify in some patients [10]. Indeed, genetic testing is generally not needed as the disease is primarily diagnosed via clinical and biochemical features [6–8, 10, 18]. A number of diagnostic criteria have been proposed [8], but they are typically based on family history (i.e., HeFH in both parents and/or premature CAD), the presence of physical manifestations (i.e., tendon xanthomas, corneal arcus) at an early age, severely increased LDL-C, and molecular diagnosis. Patients with HoFH generally have untreated LDL-C levels >500 mg/dL (>13 mmol/L) or treated levels ≥300 mg/dL (≥7.76 mmol/L) [8]. However, not all patients (especially children) with HoFH have significantly elevated LDL-C, with more than one-half of Dutch children with HoFH having LDL-C levels between 217 and 379 mg/dL (5.6–9.8 mmol/L) [10]. Patients with a suspected diagnosis of HoFH should typically be referred to a specialized center for proper comprehensive management [6, 10].

Since early detection of patients with HoFH is crucial for the prevention of CVD, targeted and cascade (i.e., identifying family members at risk) screening is recommended for the identification of new cases in adults [6, 7, 16, 19, 20]. Targeted screening to identify index cases is recommended for patients with hypercholesterolemia and at least one of the following features: personal/family history of xanthomas or premature CVD or family history of significant hypercholesterolemia or sudden premature cardiac death [6, 7]. Specific criteria in Europe (i.e., European Atherosclerosis Society [EAS]) are similar, but somewhat different than those of the National Lipid Association in the United States (US), with slightly different cholesterol cut-points for screening [21]. Such testing is important because most patients identified via screening were not aware of the diagnosis and were therefore not receiving therapy [17]. The index subject should be referred for genetic screening and a family pedigree should be created to identify potential cases, followed by cascade screening with LDL-C measurements [7]. Targeted screening is also recommended in children and adolescents with CV risk factors [6, 16]. Prenatal diagnosis is possible, and it is recommended that the partners of known cases of HeFH should be tested to exclude the disease [22]. Economic modeling has shown that comprehensive screening using cholesterol and DNA testing is cost-effective [19].

5. Treatment options

Given the severity of hypercholesterolemia with increased CV risk, HoFH requires intensive therapy. However, HoFH is often unresponsive to traditional treatment [20]. A number of societies and associations in the United States (American College of Cardiology/American Heart Association; National Lipid Association) [20, 23, 24], Europe (EAS; National Institute for Health and Care Excellence) [10, 25], and Canada (Canadian Cardiovascular Society) [6] have published guidelines on the treatment of HoFH. The primary target of treatment in these guidelines is the reduction of LDL-C via a combination of lifestyle, antihyperlipidemic pharmacotherapy, and apheresis [6, 10, 20, 23, 26]. Since lipid-lowering therapy is associated with a delayed onset of CVD and prolonged survival, early and aggressive therapy should be initiated as soon as possible [6, 10]. The EAS has recommended LDL-C targets of <100 mg/dL (<2.5 mmol/L) in children and <70 mg/dL (<1.8 mmol/L) in adults [10].

Statins, the first line of pharmacotherapy to lowering cholesterol level, effectively lower LDL-C 10% to 25% in patients with HoFH [10, 26], and even more (approximately 50% reduction of LDL-C) in those with HeFH [26]. The combination with ezetimibe (acholesterol absorption inhibitor) leads to additive 15–20% LDL-C reductions [6, 10]. Other agents such as bile acid sequestrants, niacin, fibrates, and probucol can be considered. A clinical study of HoFH patients from South Africa found that statin use was associated with a 51% reduction in the risk of major CV events and a 66% reduction in the risk of death although the mean LDL-C levels in the patients were only reduced 26% [27].

Because of very high LDL-C levels in HoFH, its target level is extremely difficult to achieve though cholesterol has been reduced [10]. The inability of standard lipid-lowering therapies to produce the necessary effect is further exacerbated by the fact that these agents work by increasing expression of LDLRs. Thus, lipoprotein apheresis should be considered in all patients with HoFH and should be initiated early. For example, the EAS guidelines recommend that apheresis should ideally be initiated by age 5 and not later than age 8 in children with HoFH [10]. Canadian guidelines recommend apheresis in adults with HoFH with LDL-C >329 mg/dL (>8.5 mmol/L) and in children (weighing >15 kg or >7 years of age) with an LDL-C >193 mg/dL (>5 mmol/L) [6]. LDL apheresis selectively removes LDL-C without affecting immunoglobulins or other proteins with reductions of approximately 60% [18]. However, a rapid rebound in LDL-C is seen with levels returning to baseline within 2 to 4 weeks [18, 20]. Although there are no randomized trials evaluating the effect of apheresis on clinical outcomes, there is clinical evidence that apheresis can contribute to regression and/or stabilization of atherosclerotic plaque [10]. Limitations to the use of apheresis include lack of availability in some locations, high cost, long procedure duration, and the need to maintain vascular access [4]. It is recommended that patients on apheresis undergo routine monitoring to assess carotid atherosclerosis (carotid ultrasound), progression of aortic valve/root disease (echocardiography), and progression of coronary atherosclerosis (stress exercise test) [6].

6. New pharmacologic therapies

Recently, three novel agents have become available—mipomersen, lomitapide, and evolocumab—each with a unique mechanism of action. Two of these agents (mipomersen and lomitapide) target very low-density lipoprotein (VLDL) production, while the other (evolocumab) causes increased catabolism of LDL-C via LDLR recycling (**Figure 2**) [10].

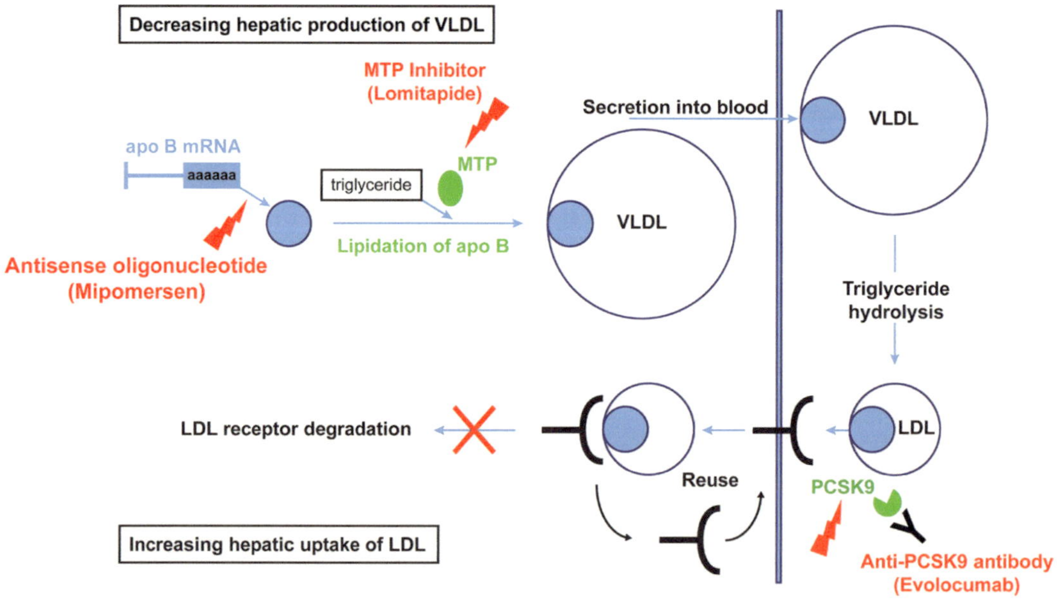

Figure 2. Mechanisms of action of mipomersen, lomitapide, and evolocumab. Modified from Cuchel et al. 2014 [10].

Properties of these agents are summarized in **Table 1** [28–32] and are discussed in detail in the following sections. These agents produce additive LDL-C lowering when combined with other lipid-lowering therapies such as statins, ezetimibe, and apheresis [10] and represent promising approaches to the treatment of HoFH for those patients who cannot achieve LDL-C targets with conventional therapy.

http://dx.doi.org/10.5772/63949

Agent	MOA	Indication	Dosage and administration	LDL-C lowering	Adverse events
Mipomersen[29]	Oligonucleotide inhibitor of apolipoprotein B-100 synthesis	Adjunctive therapy in HoFH	**HoFH:** 200 mg SC once weekly	25%	Increased transaminases Hepatic steatosis Injection-site reactions
Lomitapide [28,30,31]	Microsomal triglyceride transfer protein inhibitor	Adjunctive therapy in HoFH	**HoFH:** Initiate at 5 mg/day, titrating to max of 60 mg/day	46%	Increased transaminases Hepatic steatosis
Evolocumab[32]	PCSK9 inhibitor	Adjunctive therapy in HeFH and HoFH	**HeFH:** 140 mg SC every 2 weeks or 420 mg SC once monthly[b] **HoFH:** 420 mg SC once monthly	23%	Nasopharyngitis, upper respiratory tract infection, influenza, back pain, and injection-site reactions

[a]Based on phase III trials in HoFH;

[b]Administered as three injections consecutively within 30 minutes.

HeFH, heterozygous familial hypercholesterolemia; HoFH, homozygous familial hypercholesterolemia; LDL-C, low-density lipoprotein cholesterol; MOA, mechanisms of action; PCSK9, proprotein convertase subtilisin/kexin type 9; SC, subcutaneous.

Table 1. Novel agents for the treatment of HoFH.

6.1. Mipomersen

6.1.1. Pharmacodynamics

Apo B is the primary protein of VLDL, intermediate density lipoprotein, and LDL and is essential for the production and catabolism of VLDL and LDL [33, 34]. Apo B is involved in the packaging and distribution of both dietary and endogenously produced cholesterol and triglycerides by lipoproteins [35]. The atherosclerotic potential of apo B is evidenced by the observation that apo B concentrations are highly predictive for atherosclerotic disease, including patients with FH [8, 33].

Mipomersen is an antisense oligonucleotide against the mRNA of apo B-100, the primary ligand for the LDLR [33, 34]. The drug reduces apo B mRNA translation, and thereby the synthesis of apo B by ribosomes, resulting in a reduction in the secretion of VLDL. Thus, mipomersen targets the production of LDL rather than its clearance (**Figure 2**) [34]. In animal models, species-specific inhibition of antisense apo B leads to reductions in apo B-100, LDL-C, and total cholesterol in a dose- and time-dependent manner [29, 35].

Mipomersen is readily absorbed after subcutaneous administration with the highest drug concentrations in the liver and kidney. Bioavailability ranges from 54% to 78% over a dose range of 50 to 400 mg [29]. Elimination is primarily via metabolism by endonucleases and renal excretion (as parent drug and metabolites) and the half-life ranges from 1 to 2 months [29, 35]. In the United States, mipomersen is indicated as an adjunct to lipid-lowering medications and diet to reduce LDL-C, apo B, total cholesterol, and non-HDL-C in patients with HoFH [36]. The drug is administered once weekly by subcutaneous injection [29].

6.1.2. *Efficacy*

Based on its mechanism of action and its demonstrated activity in patients with hypercholesterolemia as either monotherapy or in combinations, it is reasonable that mipomersen would be effective in the treatment of HoFH [35]. In a phase II, open-label, study, mipomersen was administered in a dose-escalation fashion (50, 100, 200, and 300 mg) to nine patients with HoFH. Patients received five doses over 2 weeks followed by weekly dosing through week 6 ($n = 5$) or week 13 ($n = 4$). At week 6, LDL-C reductions ranged from 0.5% to 36%. By week 13, the reductions ranged from 9.0% to 51.1%[29].

The phase III trial of mipomersen in patients with HoFH included 51 patients with clinical diagnosis or genetically confirmed HoFH [37]. Mean baseline LDL-C was 402 mg/dL (10.4 mmol/L). Patients who received maximally tolerated doses of lipid-lowering drug were randomized to receive mipomersen 200 mg subcutaneously ($n = 34$) or placebo ($n = 17$) once weekly for 26 weeks [37]. The primary endpoint was the percent change in LDL-C concentration from baseline. Secondary endpoints were changes from baseline in apo B, total cholesterol, and non-HDL-C concentrations. At 26 weeks, mipomersen-treated patients achieved significant reductions in all primary and secondary endpoints versus placebo: LDL-C (–24.7%), apo B (–26.8%), total cholesterol (–21.2%), and non-HDLC (–24.5%). By comparison, reductions for those in the placebo group were: LDL-C (–3.3%), apo B (–2.5%), total cholesterol (–2.0%), and non-HDL-C (–2.9%). In addition, mipomersen was also associated with substantial reductions in Lp(a) (–31.1%), triglycerides (–17.4%), and VLDL (–17.4%), and a significant increase in HDL-C (+15.1%). Notably, there was substantial variability in the reduction of LDL-C concentrations among HoFH patients receiving mipomersen with values ranging from +2% to –82%. The magnitude of treatment effect was independent of baseline LDL-C, age, race, or sex in multivariate analysis [37].

6.1.3. *Safety/tolerability*

In the phase III HoFH trial, the most common adverse events among patients with HoFH were injection-site reactions (76%), flu-like symptoms (29%), nausea (18%), headache (15%), and chest pain (12%). Injection-site reactions included erythema (56%), hematoma (35%), pain (35%), pruritus (29%), discoloration (29%), macule (15%), papule (12%), and swelling (12%). Similar rates of injection-site reactions were observed in pooled data from other clinical trials with rates of 84% and 33%, respectively, for those in the mipomersen and placebo groups [29]. Most reactions were of mild to moderate severity with only 5% discontinuing treatment because of an injection-site reaction. In pooled phase III trials that included all patients with hypercholesterolemia, 30% of patients experienced flu-like symptoms (e.g., pyrexia, chills, myalgia, arthralgia, malaise, fatigue) compared with 16% of those receiving placebo [29].

Laboratory abnormalities in the phase III HoFH trial were primarily characterized by elevated liver transaminases. Alanine aminotransferase (ALT) increases of ≥1 but ≤3 times the upper limit of normal (ULN) were observed in 50% of patients in the mipomersen groups but was similar to that seen with placebo (53%). However, increased ALT of ≥3 × ULN was seen in 12% of mipomersen-treated patients but none of the placebo-treated patients [37]. In the pooled phase III trials, 8.4% of patients receiving mipomersen experienced an elevated ALT >3 × ULN on two consecutive occasions at least 7 days apart compared to 0.0% of placebo-treated patients [29]. These ALT changes were generally associated with lesser elevations of aspartate aminotransferase (AST). Mipomersen was also associated with an increase in hepatic fat in 9.6% of patients compared with 0.02% of placebo-treated patients. However, this increase was not accompanied by changes in patient weight, plasma glucose, or HbA1c, suggesting that there is no associated increased risk of metabolic syndrome. It is suggested that the hepatic steatosis and elevated transaminase concentrations are inherent consequences of attenuating apo B production. Nevertheless, mipomersen carries a black box warning for the risk of hepatotoxicity (i.e., increased transaminases and hepatic steatosis) and the drug is only available in the United States via a Risk Evaluation and Mitigation Strategy program [29].

6.2. Lomitapide

6.2.1. Pharmacodynamics

The microsomal triglyceride transfer protein (MTP) is an intracellular lipid-transfer protein located in the lumen of the endoplasmic reticulum. It is responsible for binding and moving individual lipid molecules between membranes. MTP is a major mediator of the assembly and secretion of apo B-containing lipoproteins such as VLDL from the liver, which is converted into LDL-C, and chylomicrons, which contain dietary cholesterol and triglycerides, from the intestine [30, 31, 38]. The rare genetic condition abetalipoproteinemia provides insight into the importance of MTP in lipid handling and transport. Abetalipoproteinemia is characterized by loss-of-function mutations in the gene encoding MTP (i.e., *MTTP*) and is associated with marked hypocholesterolemia and an absence of apo B-containing lipoproteins in the plasma [35]. Lack of functional MTP in abetalipoproteinemia results in the inability to load apo B with lipoproteins and the targeted proteasomal degradation of apo B. This leads to a loss of intestinal secretion of chylomicrons and liver secretion of VLDL and a consequent lack of LDL-C in the plasma [35]. Thus, inhibition of MTP is a potentially powerful therapeutic target to reduce the production of apo B-containing lipoproteins, particularly VLDL (the precursor of LDL-C) [30].

Lomitapide is a small molecule that inhibits MTP action. By binding directly to MTP, lomitapide inhibits the synthesis of triglyceride-rich chylomicrons in the intestine and VLDL in the liver, with a resulting reduction in plasma LDL-C [39]. The mechanism of action of lomitapide in inhibiting MTP is illustrated in **Figure 2**.

Oral absorption of lomitapide is poor with an absolute bioavailability of 7%, thought to be due to a first-pass effect. Lomitapide pharmacokinetics is approximately dose proportional after single oral doses of 10–100 mg. The drug is extensively metabolized in the liver and has a terminal half-life of 39.7 hours [28, 30]. Lomitapide is indicated in the United States and the European Union as an adjunct to a low-fat diet and other lipid-lowering treatments, including LDL apheresis where available, to reduce LDL-C, total cholesterol, apo B, and non-HDL-C in patients with HoFH [28, 39].

6.2.2. Efficacy

An initial study in 18 patients with HoFH evaluated the addition of lomitapide to usual lipid-lowering therapy, including apheresis [40]. The dose of lomitapide was gradually titrated during the first 14–18 weeks to a target dose of 60 mg/day (80 mg/day if LDL and safety criteria were met). The mean overall LDL-C reduction was 44% at 6 months compared with baseline but the individual values ranged from an increase in LDL-C of 19% to a reduction of 93%, indicating a wide variability of effect. Four patients achieved an LDL-C <100 mg/dL (<2.6 mmol/L) and another two achieved levels <170 mg/dL (<4.4 mmol/L) [40].

The pivotal phase III open-label trial included 29 patients with HoFH based on clinical criteria or documented genetic mutations [41]. Upon enrollment, patients were required to enter a 6-week run-in phase in which patients were initiated on concomitant lipid-lowering therapy (including apheresis), vitamin E, essential fatty acids, and a low-fat diet. Patients then entered a 26-week efficacy phase where lomitapide was initiated at 5 mg/day and titrated (at 4-week intervals) up to a maximum of 60 mg/day. Following the efficacy phase, patients continued lomitapide therapy in a 52-week safety phase. Mean baseline total cholesterol and LDL-C levels were 429 mg/dL (11.1 mmol/L) and 336 mg/dL (8.7 mmol/L), respectively [41]. Twenty-three of 29 patients completed both the efficacy phase (26 weeks) and safety phase (52 weeks). At the end of 26 weeks, patients achieved statistically significant mean reductions from baseline in total cholesterol (–46%; $P < 0.0001$) and LDL-C (–50%; $P < 0.0001$) [41]. The large majority of patients ($n = 19/23$ [83%]) achieved LDL-C reductions >25% and one-half ($n = 12/23$) had a >50% reduction [41]. Furthermore, 8 patients achieved LDL-C concentrations <100 mg/dL (<2.6 mmol/L). Based on these LDL-C reductions, three patients permanently discontinued apheresis and three permanently increased the time interval between apheresis treatments. Significant reductions from baseline were also seen for VLDL cholesterol (–45%), non-HDL-C (–50%), triglycerides (–45%), and apo B (–49%). Lipid lowering was independent of the use of apheresis, suggesting that apheresis does not affect the lipid-lowering efficacy of lomitapide [42]. These reductions were maintained throughout the 52-week safety phase with reductions of 35% and 38%, respectively, for total cholesterol and LDL-C despite changes in concomitant lipid-lowering therapy [41]. Nineteen of the 23 patients who competed the efficacy and safety phases entered a long-term extension study [43, 44]. As of 2015, the median duration of treatment was 5.1 years [43]. At 126 weeks, mean LDL-C levels were reduced by 46%. Similar

http://dx.doi.org/10.5772/63949

reductions were also observed in apo B (–54%), non-HDL-C (–47%), VLDL cholesterol (–37%), and triglycerides (–38%) [43, 44].

Additional evidence of the efficacy of lomitapide in HoFH comes from a Japanese trial [45] and the Lomitapide Observational Worldwide Evaluation Registry (LOWER) [45, 46]. The Japanese trial included nine patients with a mean baseline LDL-C of 199 mg/dL (5.2 mmol/L), which was reduced to 118 mg/dL (3.1 mmol/L) at week 26 (–42%) [45]. Significant reductions were also seen for total cholesterol (–32%), non-HDL-C (–40%), VLDL (–42%), apo B (–45%), and triglycerides (–42%) [45]. LOWER is a noninterventional registry open to lomitapide-treated patients that is designed to evaluate the long-term safety and efficacy of lomitapide in clinical practice and is eventually expected to enroll at least 300 patients and follow them for at least 10 years [47]. As of March 2015, 84 patients had enrolled in LOWER, with all but one from the United States [46]. Titration of lomitapide occurred slower than in the pivotal phase III trial, with a mean dose of 10 mg reached only after 12 months. The mean reduction in LDL-C at month 4 was 42%, with 38% of patients achieving a reduction of at least 50% at 6 months [46, 47].

6.2.3. *Safety/tolerability*

Oral lomitapide was generally well tolerated in patients with HoFH. Although the majority of patients experienced an adverse event in the phase III trial (n = 27/29 [93%] in the efficacy phase; n = 21/23 [91%] in the safety phase), most events were mild to moderate in intensity [41]. The most common adverse events were gastrointestinal in nature, with 27/29 patients in the efficacy phase and 21/23 patients in the safety phase experiencing a gastrointestinal event [41]. The most common events in the phase III trial were gastrointestinal in nature (27 patients during the efficacy phase and 17 during the safety phase), most commonly manifested as diarrhea, nausea, dyspepsia, and vomiting [41, 43]. Three patients discontinued treatment due to a gastrointestinal event [41]. The incidence of gastrointestinal events decreased during the extension phase: diarrhea (42%), nausea (32%), vomiting (26%), and dyspepsia (11%) [43].

Ten patients in the phase III trial had elevated levels of ALT, AST, or both >3 × ULN at least once during the trial, and four patients had elevations at least 5 × ULN [41]. No patient discontinued treatment permanently because of these elevations and all were managed by either dose reduction or temporary interruption of lomitapide [41, 43]. In the LOWER registry, elevated transaminase levels ≥3 × ULN were observed in only 16 patients (19%) [46].

Among the 20 patients from the phase III trials with evaluable nuclear magnetic resonance spectroscopy data, hepatic fat increased from 1% at baseline to 8.6% at the end of week 26 and 8.3% at week 78 [41]. Hepatic fat continued to increase through the extension trial [43], although the accumulation of fat appears to be reversible after discontinuation of lomitapide [39]. Whether this fat accumulation is a risk factor for the development of steatohepatitis and cirrhosis is currently unknown. No cases of cirrhosis or late-stage liver disease have been identified in the long-term extension studies [43].

6.3. Evolocumab

6.3.1. Pharmacodynamics

PCSK9 is a key regulator of LDLR function. When PCSK9 binds to the LDLR, LDLR degradation is enhanced in the liver, thereby increasing LDL-C plasma concentrations [4].Although some patients with HoFH have no LDLR function, up to 75% have residual activity (between 2% and 25%) [2]. Patients with HoFH also have increased PCSK9 function. Among patients with residual LDLR function, PCSK9 inhibition may be useful for lowering LDL-C [2]. Evolocumab is a human immunoglobulin G2 monoclonal antibody directed against human PCSK9. By binding to PCSK9, evolocumab inhibits circulating PCSK9 from binding to the LDLR, preventing PCSK9-mediated LDLR degradation and permitting LDLR to recycle back to the liver cell surface. This increases the number of LDLRs available to clear LDL from the blood, thereby lowering LDL-C level (**Figure 2**) [32, 48, 49].

6.3.2. Efficacy

The addition of evolocumab to stable lipid-lowering therapy was evaluated in an open-label pilot trial in eight patients with LDLR-negative or LDLR-defective HoFH [32]. Patients received subcutaneous evolocumab 420 mg every 4 weeks for 12 weeks, maintained for an additional 12 weeks at 4-week intervals, and then 420 mg of evolocumab every 2 weeks for an additional 12 weeks [32]. All eight patients had LDLR mutations, with six patients having defective receptor status (i.e., residual LDLR function) and two having negative LDLR function. Mean baseline LDL-C was 441 mg/dL (11.4 mmol/L) [32]. After 12 weeks of every 4-week dosing, mean LDL-C decreased by a mean of 17% (range, +5% to –44%). The two patients with negative LDLR activity did not achieve reductions in LDL-C [32]. After 12 weeks of every 2-week dosing, mean LDL-C was reduced by 14%, again with no reductions in the two patients that were LDLR-negative. Apo B was reduced by 14.9% and 12.5% by the 4-week and 2-week dosing schedules and Lp(a) was reduced by 11.7% and 18.6%, respectively, by the two schedules. However, there was little change in triglycerides, HDL-C, or apolipoprotein A1 with either schedule [32].

The pivotal randomized, phase III, double-blind, placebo-controlled trial included 49 patients with HoFH on stable lipid-lowering therapy (but not apheresis) for at least 4 weeks. Patients were randomized in a 2:1 ratio to receive evolocumab 420 mg or placebo every 4 weeks [48]. LDLR mutations in both alleles were present in 45 of 48 patients (94%), with 22 of these having the same mutation in both alleles (true HoFH) and 23 having different mutations in each LDLR allele (i.e., compound heterozygous FH) [48]. One patient receiving evolocumab had LDLR receptor-negative mutations in both alleles and another had autosomal recessive hypercholesterolemia. The mean decrease in ultracentrifugation LDL-C was 23.1% for those receiving evolocumab compared with a 7.9% increase for the placebo group (primary endpoint) [48]. Evolocumab was also associated with a 19.2% reduction in apo B at week 12, although changes in Lp(a), HDL-C, and triglycerides were not significantly different relative to placebo [48]. Response to evolocumab correlated with the underlying genetic cause of HoFH, with a greater reduction in LDL-C among those with two LDLR-defective mutations than in those with even

http://dx.doi.org/10.5772/63949

a single LDLR-negative mutation. However, among the 20 patients receiving evolocumab who had defects in either one or both alleles, a 29.5% reduction in ultracentrifugation LDL-C was achieved [48]. The patient with LDLR-negative mutations in both alleles and the one with autosomal recessive hypercholesterolemia did not respond to evolocumab (LDL-C levels increased by 3–10%) [48].

The efficacy of evolocumab in combination with apheresis is under evaluation in the Trial Assessing Long Term Use of PCSK9 Inhibition in Subjects with Genetic LDL Disorders (TAUSSIG) in patients with severe FH not controlled with current lipid therapy [50]. Patients received evolocumab 420 mg and apheresis every 2 weeks. An interim analysis found that evolocumab was associated with a mean reduction of 17% in LDL-C at week 12 (n = 24) and 20% at week 24 (n = 12) [50]. Four patients were able to stop or decrease the frequency of apheresis. The three patients with LDLR-negative mutations in both alleles did not respond to evolocumab. Evolocumab is indicated in the United States and EU as an adjunct to diet and other LDL-lowering therapies for the treatment of patients with HoFH who require additional lowering of LDL-C.

6.3.3. *Safety/tolerability*

In the phase III trial in patients with HoFH, the most common adverse events among those receiving evolocumab were upper respiratory tract infection (9%), influenza (9%), gastroenteritis (6%), nasopharyngitis (6%), and increased ALT or AST ≥3 × ULN [48]. There were no adverse event-related treatment discontinuations. These rates of adverse events are generally consistent with those seen in other large randomized trials evaluating evolocumab in the treatment of hypercholesterolemia [49]. Immunogenicity appears to be uncommon, with only 0.1% of patients in pooled clinical trials testing positive for binding antibody development. There was no evidence of neutralizing antibodies and no evidence that the presence of antidrug antibodies impacted the pharmacokinetic profile, clinical response, or safety of evolocumab [49].

7. Conclusions

HoFH is a rare disease that is underdiagnosed and undertreated and is associated with substantial morbidity and mortality. Early diagnosis and aggressive therapy are the cornerstones of the management of HoFH. Until recently, therapeutic options were limited and insufficient to get patients to their treatment goals. The availability of novel pharmacologic agents provides clinicians with additional treatment options in this difficult-to-treat population. **Figure 3** summarizes the suggested treatment algorithm of the EAS for patients with HoFH [10].

This algorithm highlights the novel treatment options that will allow greater reductions in lipid levels in HoFH patients and let them achieve their target goals. It is hoped and expected that these expanded options will ultimately translate into improvements in clinical outcomes including a decrease in CV events and CVD-related mortality.

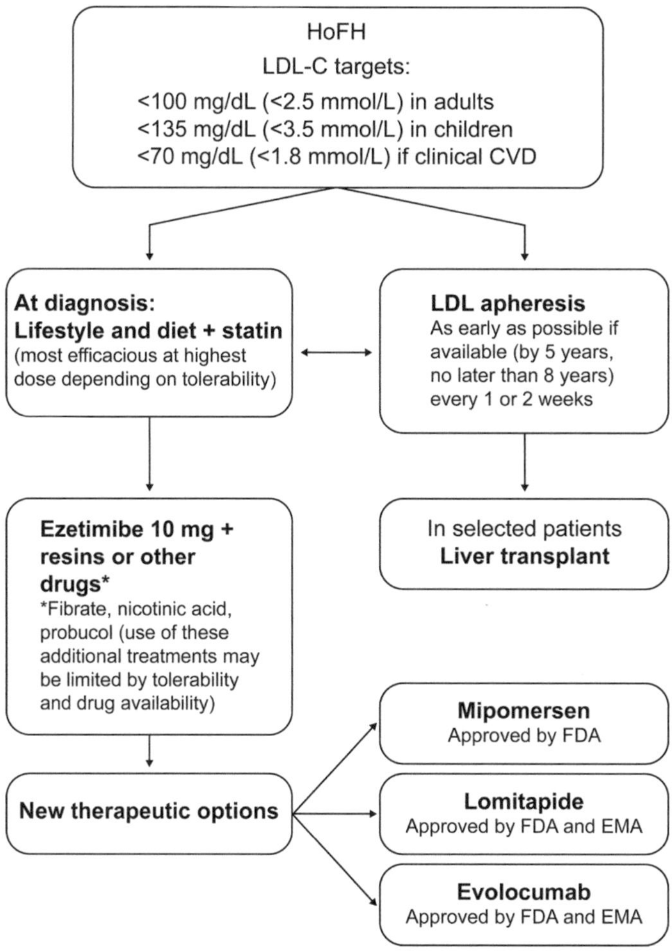

Figure 3. European Atherosclerosis Society treatment algorithm for the management of HoFH. Modified from Cuchel et al. 2014 [10].

Author details

Min-Ji Charng

Address all correspondence to: mjcharng@vghtpe.gov.tw

Division of Cardiology, Taipei Veterans General Hospital and National Yang-Ming University, Taipei, Taiwan, R.O.C.

References

[1] Sniderman AD, Tsimikas S, Fazio S. The severe hypercholesterolemia phenotype: clinical diagnosis, management, and emerging therapies. J Am Coll Cardiol. 2014;63:1935–1947.

[2] Chiou KR, Charng MJ. Genetic diagnosis of familial hypercholesterolemia in Han J Clin Lipidol. 2016;10:490–496.

[3] Marais AD, Blom DJ. Recent advances in the treatment of homozygous familial hypercholesterolaemia. Curr Opin Lipidol. 2013;24:288–294.

[4] Farnier M, Bruckert E. Severe familial hypercholesterolaemia: current and future management. Arch Cardiovasc Dis. 2012;105:656–665.

[5] Singh S, Bittner V. Familial hypercholesterolemia—epidemiology, diagnosis, and screening. Curr Atheroscler Rep. 2015;17:482–485.

[6] Genest J, Hegele RA, Bergeron J, Brophy J, Carpentier A, Couture P, et al. Canadian Cardiovascular Society position statement on familial hypercholesterolemia. Can J Cardiol. 2014;30:1471–1481.

[7] Nordestgaard BG, Chapman MJ, Humphries SE, Ginsberg HN, Masana L, Descamps OS, et al. Familial hypercholesterolaemia is underdiagnosed and undertreated in the general population: guidance for clinicians to prevent coronary heart disease: consensus statement of the European Atherosclerosis Society. Eur Heart J. 2013;34:3478–3490.

[8] Raal FJ, Santos RD. Homozygous familial hypercholesterolemia: current perspectives on diagnosis and treatment. Atherosclerosis. 2012;223:262–268.

[9] Horton JD, Cohen JC, Hobbs HH. PCSK9: a convertase that coordinates LDL catabolism. J Lipid Res. 2009;50(Suppl):S172–S177.

[10] Cuchel M, Bruckert E, Ginsberg HN, Raal FJ, Santos RD, Hegele RA, et al. Homozygous familial hypercholesterolaemia: new insights and guidance for clinicians to improve detection and clinical management. A position paper from the Consensus Panel on Familial Hypercholesterolaemia of the European Atherosclerosis Society. Eur Heart J. 2014;35:2146–2157.

[11] Fahed AC, Safa RM, Haddad FF, Bitar FF, Andary RR, Arabi MT, et al. Homozygous familial hypercholesterolemia in Lebanon: a genotype/phenotype correlation. Mol Genet Metab. 2011;102:181–188.

[12] Kusters DM, Huijgen R, Defesche JC, Vissers MN, Kindt I, Hutten BA, et al. Founder mutations in the Netherlands: geographical distribution of the most prevalent mutations in the low-density lipoprotein receptor and apolipoprotein B genes. Neth Heart J. 2011;19:175–182.

[13] Mabuchi H, Nohara A, Noguchi T, Kobayashi J, Kawashiri MA, Tada H, et al. Molecular genetic epidemiology of homozygous familial hypercholesterolemia in the Hokuriku district of Japan. Atherosclerosis. 2011;214:404–407.

[14] Moorjani S, Roy M, Gagne C, Davignon J, Brun D, Toussaint M, et al. Homozygous familial hypercholesterolemia among French Canadians in Quebec Province. Arteriosclerosis. 1989;9:211–216.

[15] Seftel HC, Baker SG, Sandler MP, Forman MB, Joffe BI, Mendelsohn D, et al. A host of hypercholesterolaemic homozygotes in South Africa. Br Med J. 1980;281:633–636.

[16] Feldman DI, Blaha MJ, Santos RD, Jones SR, Blumenthal RS, Toth PP, et al. Recommendations for the management of patients with familial hypercholesterolemia. Curr Atheroscler Rep. 2015;17:473. DOI: 10.1007/s11883-014-0473-6

[17] Alonso R, Mata P, Zambon D, Mata N, Fuentes-Jimenez F. Early diagnosis and treatment of familial hypercholesterolemia: improving patient outcomes. Expert Rev Cardiovasc Ther. 2013;11:327–342. DOI: 10.1586/erc.13.7

[18] Mombelli G, Pavanello C. Novel therapeutic strategies for the homozygous familial hypercholesterolemia. Recent Pat Cardiovasc Drug Discov. 2013;8:143–150. DOI: 10.2174/15748901112079990001

[19] Minhas R, Humphries SE, Qureshi N, Neil HA. Controversies in familial hypercholesterolaemia: recommendations of the NICE Guideline Development Group for the identification and management of familial hypercholesterolaemia. Heart. 2009;95:584–587. DOI: 10.1136/hrt.2008.162909

[20] Robinson JG. Management of familial hypercholesterolemia: a review of the recommendations from the National Lipid Association Expert Panel on Familial Hypercholesterolemia. J Manag Care Pharm. 2013;19:139–149.

[21] Gouni-Berthold I, Berthold HK. Familial hypercholesterolemia: etiology, diagnosis and new treatment options. Curr Pharm Des. 2014;20:6220–6229.

[22] Reiner Z, Catapano AL, De Backer G, Graham I, Taskinen MR, Wiklund O, et al. ESC/EAS Guidelines for the management of dyslipidaemias: the Task Force for the management of dyslipidaemias of the European Society of Cardiology (ESC) and the European Atherosclerosis Society (EAS). Eur Heart J. 2011;32:1769–1818. DOI: 10.1093/eurheartj/ehr158

[23] Ray KK, Kastelein JJ, Boekholdt SM, Nicholls SJ, Khaw KT, Ballantyne CM, et al. The ACC/AHA 2013 guideline on the treatment of blood cholesterol to reduce atherosclerotic cardiovascular disease risk in adults: the good the bad and the uncertain: a comparison with ESC/EAS guidelines for the management of dyslipidaemias 2011. Eur Heart J. 2014;35:960–968. DOI: 10.1093/eurheartj/ehu107

[24] Stone NJ, Robinson JG, Lichtenstein AH, Bairey Merz CN, Blum CB, Eckel RH, et al. 2013 ACC/AHA guideline on the treatment of blood cholesterol to reduce atheroscler-

otic cardiovascular risk in adults: a report of the American College of Cardiology/ American Heart Association Task Force on Practice Guidelines. Circulation. 2014;129:S1–S45. DOI: 10.1161/01.cir.0000437738.63853.7a

[25] National Institute on Clinical Care and Excellence (NICE). Familial hypercholesterolaemia: identifification and management.2008. Available from: http://www.nice.org.uk/guidance/cg71. [Accessed Nov 23, 2015]

[26] Bruckert E. Recommendations for the management of patients with homozygous familial hypercholesterolaemia: overview of a new European Atherosclerosis Society consensus statement. Atheroscler Suppl. 2014;15:26–32.

[27] Raal FJ, Pilcher GJ, Panz VR, van Deventer HE, Brice BC, Blom DJ, et al. Reduction in mortality in subjects with homozygous familial hypercholesterolemia associated with advances in lipid-lowering therapy. Circulation. 2011;124:2202–2207.

[28] JUXTAPID (lomitapide): package insert. Cambridge, MA: Aegerion Pharmaceuticals, Inc.; 2015.

[29] McGowan MP, Moriarty PM, Backes JM. The effects of mipomersen, a second-generation antisense oligonucleotide, on atherogenic (apoB-containing) lipoproteins in the treatment of homozygous familial hypercholesterolemia. Clin Lipidol. 2014;9:487–503.

[30] Perry CM. Lomitapide: a review of its use in adults with homozygous familial hypercholesterolemia. Am J Cardiovasc Drugs. 2013;13:285–296.

[31] Raal FJ. Lomitapide for homozygous familial hypercholesterolaemia. Lancet. 2013;381:7–8.

[32] Stein EA, Honarpour N, Wasserman SM, Xu F, Scott R, Raal FJ. Effect of the proprotein convertase subtilisin/kexin 9 monoclonal antibody, AMG 145, in homozygous familial hypercholesterolemia. Circulation. 2013;128:2113–2120.

[33] Parhofer KG. Mipomersen: evidence-based review of its potential in the treatment of homozygous and severe heterozygous familial hypercholesterolemia. Core Evid. 2012;7:29–38.

[34] Patel N, Hegele RA. Mipomersen as a potential adjunctive therapy for hypercholesterolemia. Expert Opin Pharmacother. 2010;11:2569–2572.

[35] Rader DJ, Kastelein JJ. Lomitapide and mipomersen: two first-in-class drugs for reducing low-density lipoprotein cholesterol in patients with homozygous familial hypercholesterolemia. Circulation. 2014;129:1022–1032.

[36] KYNAMRO (mipomersen sodium): package insert. Cambridge, MA: Genzyme Corporation; 2015.

[37] Raal FJ, Santos RD, Blom DJ, Marais AD, Charng MJ, Cromwell WC, et al. Mipomersen, an apolipoprotein B synthesis inhibitor, for lowering of LDL cholesterol concentrations

in patients with homozygous familial hypercholesterolaemia: a randomised, double-blind, placebo-controlled trial. Lancet. 2010;375:998–1006.

[38] Liao W, Hui TY, Young SG, Davis RA. Blocking microsomal triglyceride transfer protein interferes with apoB secretion without causing retention or stress in the ER. J Lipid Res. 2003;44:978–985.

[39] Lyseng-Willliamson KA, Perry CM. Lomitapide: a guide to its use in adults with homozygous familial hypercholesterolaemia in the EU. Drugs Ther Perspect. 2013;29:373–378.

[40] Cuchel M, Meagher E, Marais AD, Blom DJ, Theron HD, Baer AL, et al. Abstract 1077: a phase III study of microsomal triglyceride transfer protein inhibitor lomitapide (AEGR-733) in patients with homozygous familial hypercholesterolemia: interim results at 6 months [Abstract]. Circulation. 2009;120:S441.

[41] Cuchel M, Meagher EA, du Toit Theron H, Blom DJ, Marais AD, Hegele RA, et al. Efficacy and safety of a microsomal triglyceride transfer protein inhibitor in patients with homozygous familial hypercholesterolaemia: a single-arm, open-label, phase 3 study. Lancet. 2013;381:40–46.

[42] Averna M, Cuchel M, Meagher E, Du H, Theron T, Blom DJ, et al. Apheresis treatment does not affect the lipid-lowering efficacy of lomitapide, a microsomal triglyceride transfer protein inhibitor, in patients with homozygous familial hypercholesterolemia (HoFH). In: Deutschen Atherosklerosekongress 2012; 7–8 December 2012; Munich, Germany. Perfusion. 2012.

[43] Blom DJ, Averna M, Meagher E, Theron H, Sirtori C, Hegele RA, et al. Long-term efficacy and safety of lomitapide for the treatment of homozygous familial hypercholesterolemia: results of the phase 3 extension trial. In: American Heart Association; 7–11 November 2015; Orlando, FL.

[44] Cuchel M, Blom DJ, Averna MR, Meagher EA, Theron HD, Sirtori CR, et al. Sustained LDL-C lowering and stable hepatic fat levels in patients with homozygous familial hypercholesterolemia treated with the microsomal triglyceride transfer protein inhibitor, lomitapide: results of an ongoing long-term extension study [Abstract]. Circulation. 2013;128:A16516.

[45] Harada-Shiba M, Ikewaki K, Nohara A, Yanagi K, Otsubo Y, Foulds P, et al. Efficacy and safety of lomitapide in Japanese patients with homozygous familial hypercholesterolemia on cucurrent lipid-lowering therapy [Abstract]. Circulation. 2015;132:A12468.

[46] Blom DJ, Kastelein JJ, Larrey D, Makris L, Schwamiein C, Phillips H, et al. Lomitapide Observational Worldwide Evaluation Registry (LOWER): one-year data [Abstract]. Circulation. 2015;132:A10818.

[47] Blom DJ, Fayad ZA, Kastelein JJP, Larrey D, Makris L, Schwamiein C, et al. LOWER, a registry of lomitapide-treated patients with homozygous familial hypercholesterolemia: rationale and design. J Clin Lipidol. 2015;10:273–282.

[48] Raal FJ, Honarpour N, Blom DJ, Hovingh GK, Xu F, Scott R, et al. Inhibition of PCSK9 with evolocumab in homozygous familial hypercholesterolaemia (TESLA Part B): a randomised, double-blind, placebo-controlled trial. Lancet. 2015;385:341–350.

[49] REPATHA (evolocumab): package insert. Thousand Oaks, CA: Amgen, Inc.; 2015.

[50] Bruckert E, Blaha V, Stein EA, Raal FJ, Kurtz CE, Honarpour N, et al. Trial assessing long-term use of PCSK9 inhibition in patients with genetic LDL disorders (TAUSSIG): efficacy and safety in patients with homozygous familial hypercholesterolemia receiving lipid apheresis [Abstract]. Circulation. 2014;130:A17016.

Chapter 5

Cholesterol-Lowering Drugs and Therapies in Cardiovascular Disease

Zaid Almarzooq and Parmanand Singh

Additional information is available at the end of the chapter

http://dx.doi.org/10.5772/64762

Abstract

Dyslipidemia is a major risk factor for cardiovascular disease (CVD). The relationship between low-density lipoprotein concentration and cardiovascular (CV) risk has been well established in numerous epidemiological studies. The benefit of cholesterol-lowering agents has been demonstrated in patients with known CVD. On the other hand, in patients without known CVD the decision to start therapy depends on their 10-year risk prediction of CV events. 3-Hydroxy-3-methylglutaryl-coenzyme A (HMG-CoA) reductase inhibitors ("statins"), a mainstay of cholesterol-lowering therapy, have been shown to reduce both CV events and all-cause mortality. Other lipid-lowering measures (both pharmacological and nonpharmacological) have also been demonstrated in clinical trials to reduce CV outcomes. In this chapter, we review contemporary therapies used to treat dyslipidemia and discuss future directions including novel agents on the horizon.

Keywords: cholesterol treatment, cardiovascular disease, dyslipidemia, cardiovascular risk stratification, hypercholesterolemia

1. Introduction

Atherosclerotic cardiovascular disease (CVD) affects more than 15 million Americans and is considered the leading cause of death in the United States (US) in both men and women (REF). Dyslipidemia is a major risk factor for atherosclerotic CVD [1]. We review current standard treatment of abnormal cholesterol levels and discuss future directions. Lipid-altering therapies favorably impact the lipid profile by lowering total cholesterol, low-density lipoprotein (LDL), and triglycerides (TGs), while beneficially increasing high-density lipoprotein (HDL; see **Table**

1) [2–4]. In addition, lipid-altering therapies cause a desirable shift toward less atherogenic cholesterol subparticles [5]. The benefit of lipid therapy has been borne out in studies evaluating their effects on coronary atherosclerosis regression (by angiography) and incidence of major adverse cardiovascular events (MACEs) [6–10]. The lipoprotein transport system mediates the movement of cholesterol and TG in plasma, in addition to numerous other important physiologic functions. These include transport of dietary fat absorbed in the intestines to the liver, transport of modified cholesterol to peripheral tissues for cell membrane and steroid hormone synthesis, and transport of free fatty acids that may be used for fuel [11]. Lipoproteins are typically classified by their size and density. The main lipoprotein carriers of cholesterol to peripheral tissues are LDL particles. They are internalized by LDL receptors, where they are then hydrolyzed. This is an important pathway in controlling plasma cholesterol levels, as evidenced in those with loss-of-function mutations of LDL receptors leading to an inherited hyperlipidemia [12]. Importantly, LDL particles vary in size. Those with fewer cholesteryl esters and more TGs are smaller, denser, and thus more atherogenic [11].

Drug class	**LDL (%)**	**HDL (%)**	**TG (%)**
Bile acid sequestrants	↓ 15–30	↑ 3–5	No change
Cholesterol absorption inhibitors (Ezetimibe)	↓ 17–22	↑ 2–5	↓ 4–11
Fibrates	↓ 5–20	↑ 10–20	↓ 20–50
Nicotinic acid (niacin)	↓ 5–25	↑ 15–35	↓ 20–50
PCSK9 inhibitors	↓ 61–62	↑ 5–7	↓ 13–17
HMG-CoA reductase inhibitors (Statins)	↓ 18–55	↑ 5–15	↓ 7–30

Abbreviations: LDL, low-density lipoprotein cholesterol; HDL, high-density lipoprotein; TC, total cholesterol; TG, triglycerides.

Table 1. Potencies of various lipid lowering agents.

Increased concentrations of LDL have been shown in epidemiological studies to be associated with an increased risk of MACE. This was demonstrated in The Lipid Research Clinics Prevalence Study, where after 10 years of follow-up in patients with known coronary heart disease (CHD), a higher death rate was evident in those with higher levels of plasma total cholesterol and LDL [13]. In addition, those with inherited hyperlipidemia have early atherothrombosis [14]. Reducing LDL cholesterol is strongly linked to reductions in MACE, especially when using statins [10]. One-third of all middle-aged or older adults in the general population of the US and United Kingdom (UK) have an indication for statin therapy [15]. Notably decreased LDL and raising HDL levels have been associated with regression of atherosclerosis as evident in the Regression Growth Evaluation Statin Study (REGRESS) trial and several other trials [6–9].

Until recently, it was strongly recommended to treat to specific LDL targets [16]. These targets were based on post hoc analyses demonstrating greater reductions in MACE with LDL levels below certain levels. However, subsequent head-to-head statin trials compared different agents at different doses. These studies did not investigate the effects of different LDL target levels [17]. For such reasons, the most recent US guidelines advocate for using high-intensity statins for patients at high risk of cardiovascular events. By contrast, guidelines in Europe and Canada have maintained their recommendation on using LDL targets [18].

Statins are well known for pleotropic effects independent of cholesterol lowering, mainly anti-inflammatory properties [19]. In many statin trials, subjects with the largest reduction in high-sensitivity C-reactive protein (hsCRP) have decreased primary end points [20, 21]. In two statin trials, lower hsCRP and LDL levels were associated with a decrease in atheroma progression as assessed by serial intravascular ultrasound observation [22, 23]. Moreover, in the Justification for the Use of Statins in Prevention (JUPITER) trial, a decrease in MACE and all-cause mortality was seen in asymptomatic subjects with baseline elevated hsCRP levels and already low LDL level, which contemporary risk calculators would exclude from therapy. Notably, elevated LDL cholesterol is associated with MACE without the need for overt evidence of inflammation [24] .

1.1. Cardiovascular risk stratification: Who to treat?

In patients with known CVD, treatment with statins has been shown to reduce CV events and all-cause mortality, while other lipid-lowering agents have also been shown to reduce the incidence of CV events in patients not on statins [25–33]. However, in patients without known CVD, cholesterol-lowering agents have only been shown to be beneficial in those at a high risk of CV events. The absolute benefit of treatment is proportional to the underlying absolute CV risk. Therefore, it is important to target patients at a high risk of CV events rather than a specific LDL.

Various CV risk calculators have been used to identify patients at high risk. These calculators are modeled to a particular population; therefore, the choice of which risk calculator to use is important. Below, we will discuss the benefits and pitfalls of using risk calculators to guide decision to treat. The Framingham Risk score is a risk calculator based on a population from the northeastern US (https://www.framinghamheartstudy.org/risk-functions/cardiovascular-disease/10-year-risk.php#). The most current version includes major CV outcomes, stroke, and heart failure. Notably, statins have shown to reduce the incidence of major CV outcomes and stroke, but not heart failure [34]. The American Heart Association/American College of Cardiology (AHA/ACC) Pooled Cohort Equations Cardiovascular risk calculator (ASCVD) is based on a population of non-Hispanic whites and African Americans in the US (http://tools.acc.org/ASCVD-Risk-Estimator/). Compared to the Framingham risk calculator, it predicts major CV outcomes that are reduced by statins. Limitations of the ASCVD include its dichotomization of diabetes mellitus without considering its duration or type. It also does not take into account family history of premature CV disease, thus underestimating CV risk in those with significant family history of CV events [35].

The Joint British Societies (JBS-3) guidelines calculator is based on a population from the UK (http://www.jbs3risk.com/JBS3Risk.swf). In those with a low 10-year risk of CV events, the JBS-3 recommends using the QRISK® lifetime CV risk calculator [36]. Both the ASCVD and

JBS-3 predict both 10-year risk and lifetime risk of CV events. Without the data with long-term effects of statins, there is a limitation to use lifetime risk prediction for using cholesterol-lowering agents. Therefore, the use of the 10-year risk predictions has been recommended when making such decisions. In patient with diabetes, the UK Prospective Diabetes Study calculator incorporates factors important to those with diabetics that are not found in the ASCVD calculator such as diabetes duration and type [37].

Another factor used when making the decision to treat on a population-based approach is cost-effectiveness. The 2013 AHA/ACC guidelines have recommended the use of a 10-year risk of CV events threshold of 7.5% when deciding to use cholesterol-lowering agents. This was found to be more cost-effective when compared with ≥10% threshold [38].

In older patients, over age 65, the decision to treat is also influenced by the presence of other comorbidities not taken into account in the calculators above. For example, a patient with a concurrent illness with high mortality, such as metastatic pancreatic cancer, is unlikely to benefit from a cholesterol-lowering agent. Thus, clinical trials of cholesterol-lowering agents have typically excluded older patients. However, a healthy elderly patient may potentially benefit from these therapies, and in fact the absolute number to treat is much lower in a healthy elderly population, given the dramatic increase in absolute risk of CV disease in this cohort [39]. A barrier to using cholesterol-lowering agents in the elderly has been the notion that it takes years to see the benefit of cholesterol-lowering agents; however, many studies have shown that they can be beneficial in as early as 6 months, as seen in the 4S trial [40].

2. Pharmacological therapies

2.1. Statins

Statins have been shown to be beneficial in hypercholesterolemia for both primary and secondary prevention of CV events (see **Figure 1**) [41]. Their main mechanism of action involves competitive inhibition of an enzyme, 3-Hydroxy-3-methylglutaryl-coenzyme A (HMG-CoA) reductase, a rate-limiting step in cholesterol synthesis (see **Figure 2**) [42, 43]. This prevents substrate from binding to the enzymatic active site resulting in a decrease in intra-hepatic cholesterol synthesis [44]. The decrease in intrahepatic cholesterol leads to an increase in LDL receptors, and consequently an increase in LDL reuptake [45]. Other mechanisms described include alteration of hepatic Apolipoprotein B (Apo-B) secretion leading to a reduction in very low-density lipoprotein (VLDL) through decreased secretion and increased clearance. This consequently also contributes to the reduction in plasma TG [46]. Statins' effect on HDL has been attributed to their impact on hepatic microRNA33 (miR33) and consequent macrophage ATP-binding cassette transporter (ABCA)1-mediated efflux [47]. These additional mechanisms are thought to translate into clinical benefit through varied pathways including reversal of endothelial dysfunction, atheroma stabilization, and decreased thrombogenicity [48].

http://dx.doi.org/10.5772/64762

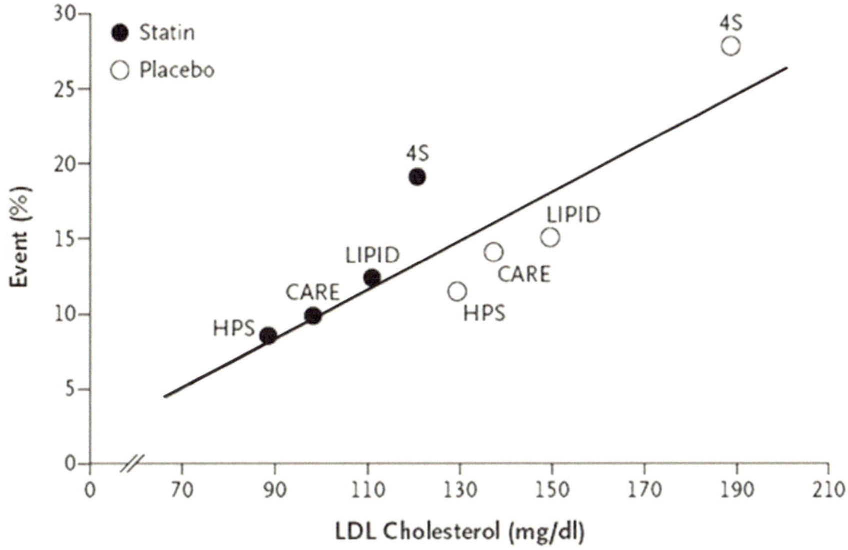

Figure 1. LDL, statins, and cardiovascular events. Reduction in cardiovascular event rates by lower low-density lipoprotein using statins in secondary prevention trials. *Abbreviations*: 4S, Scandinavian Simvastatin Survival Study; CARE, Cholesterol and Recurrent Events Trial; HPS, Heart Protection Study; LIPID, Long-term Intervention with Pravastatin in Ischemic Disease.

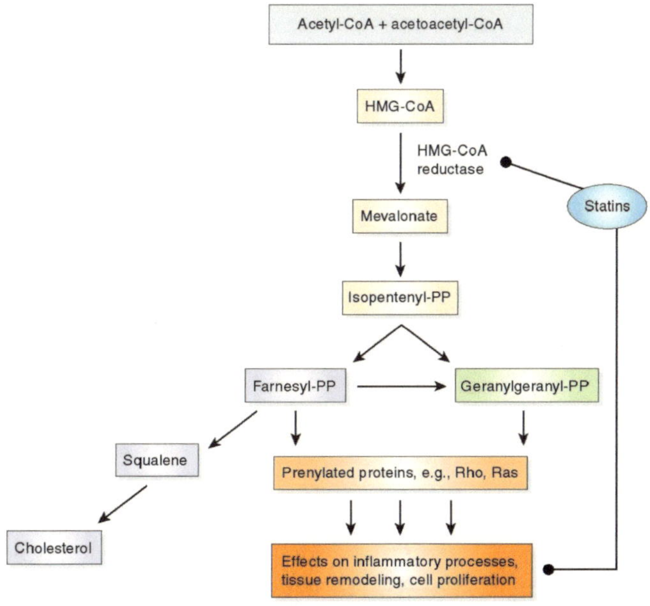

Figure 2. Mechanisms of HMG-CoA reductase inhibitors. Statins inhibit hepatic HMG-CoA reductase resulting in decreased downstream cholesterol production.

Statins are considered the most potent agents for lowering LDL cholesterol, and do so up to 63% [49]. They do have a predominant effect on small LDL particles leading to a shift in the LDL subfractions toward less atherogenic LDL [50]. Rosuvastatin has been shown to increase HDL by about 10%, appearing to be the most effective statins on HDL modification [51]. Regarding lowering TG, atorvastatin and rosuvastatin appear to be the most potent of the statins, with a dose-dependent decrease in TG of up to 33% [51].

Statins as a drug category demonstrate varying cholesterol-lowering potencies (see **Table 2**) [51–53]. Low-potency statins include simvastatin, lovastatin, pravastatin, and fluvastatin [51]. High-potency statins include atorvastatin and rosuvastatin [51]. Statins combined with a cholesterol absorption inhibitor (such as ezetimibe) or bile acid sequestrant show an additive cholesterol-lowering effect [54, 55].

Statin	TC (%)	LDL (%)	HDL (%)	TG (%)	Dose range (mg)
Atorvastatin	↓ 27–39	↓ 37–51	↑ 2–6	↓ 20–28	10–80
Rosuvastatin	↓ 33–40	↓ 46–55	↑ 8–10	↓ 20–26	10–40
Simvastatin	↓ 20–28	↓ 28–39	↑ 5–6	↓ 12–15	10–40
Pravastatin	↓ 15–22	↓ 20–30	↑ 3–6	↓ 8–13	10–40
Fluvastatin	↓ 13–19	↓ 17–23	↑ 1–3	↓ 5–13	20–80
Pitavastatin	↓ 22–31	↓ 31–44	↑ 1–4	↓ 13–22	1–4

Abbreviations: NNT, number needed to treat; WOSCOPS, West of Scotland Coronary Prevention Study; AFCAPS/TEXCAPS, Air Force/Texas Coronary Atherosclerosis Prevention Study; ALLHAT-LLT, Antihypertensive and Lipid-Lowering Treatment to Prevent Heart Attack Trial; CARDS, Collaborative Atorvastatin Diabetes Study; MEGA, Management of Elevated Cholesterol in the Primary Prevention Group of Adult Japanese; JUPITER, Justification for the Use of statins in Prevention: an Intervention Trial Evaluating Rosuvastatin; 4S, Scandinavian Simvastatin Survival Study; CARE, Cholesterol and Recurrent Events trial; LIPID, Long-Term Intervention with Pravastatin in Ischemic Disease study;. HPS, Heart Protection Study; PROSPER, Prospective Study of Pravastatin in the Elderly at Risk; PROVE-IT, Pravastatin or Atorvastatin Evaluation and Infection Therapy; TNT, Treating to New Targets; IDEAL, Incremental Decrease in End Points through Aggressive Lipid Lowering.

Table 2. Potencies of different statins.

Numerous clinical trials have shown a trend toward improved CV outcomes, but not all have demonstrated statistical significance [56]. Statins have been shown to be effective in primary prevention of CHD (see **Table 3**) 21, 25–28, 32, 41, 57–63]. This was demonstrated in the Heart Protection Study [25], CARDS trial [26], and MEGA trial [27], where statins led to a significant reduction in MACE. Statins have also been shown to be effective in the secondary prevention of CHD as well (see **Table 3**). This benefit was evident in the Scandinavian Simvastatin Survival study (4S) [28], Lipid trial [29], and MIRACLE [30], where statin use resulted in a significant reduction in MACE. In a meta-analysis, which included 17,617 patients randomized to statins from the Cholesterol and Recurrent Events (CARE), Long-term Intervention with Pravastatin in Ischemic Disease (LIPID), and 4S trials, there was a significant reduction in MACE and all-cause mortality, but no effect on noncardiovascular mortality [31]. In addition, high-dose statin therapy was shown to have a significant reduction in MACE when compared to lower-dose therapy, as seen in the Treating to New Target (TNT) trial [41] and PROVE IT-TIMI 22 trial [32].

Study	Year	Patients	Statin and daily dose	Mean baseline LDL (mg/dL)	Mean LDL reduction (%)	Reduction in coronary events (%)	NNT
Primary prevention							
WOSCOPS	1995	6595	Pravastatin 40 mg	192	26	31 ($P < 0.001$)	42
AFCAPS/TEXCAPS	1998	6605	Lovastatin 20–40 mg	150	25	37 ($P < 0.001$)	24
ALLHAT-LLT	2002	10,355	Pravastatin 40 mg	146	28	No significant reduction	
CARDS	2004	2838	Atorvastatin 10 mg	118	40	36 ($P = 0.001$)	32
MEGA	2006	7832	Pravastatin 10–20 mg	156	18	33 ($P = 0.01$)	119
JUPITER	2008	17,802	Rosuvastatin 20 mg	108	50	44 ($P <0.001$)	25
Secondary prevention							
4S	1994	4444	Simvastatin 20–40 mg	188	35	34 ($P < 0.0001$)	15
CARE	1998	4159	Pravastatin 40 mg	139	32	24 ($P = 0.003$)	33
LIPID	2002	9014	Pravastatin 40 mg	150	25	24 ($P < 0.0001$)	33
HPS	2002	20,536	Simvastatin 40 mg	3.4	1	24 ($P <0.001$)	20
PROSPER	2002	5804	Pravastatin 40 mg	147	34	14($P = 0.014$)	47
PROVE-IT	2004	4162	Atorvastatin 80 mg versus Pravastatin 40 mg	106	41	16 ($P = 0.005$)	25
TNT	2005	10,003	Atorvastatin 80 mg versus Atorvastatin 10 mg	97	21	22 ($P <0.001$)	46
IDEAL	2005	8888	Atorvastatin 80 mg versus Simvastatin 20 mg	121	34	No significant reduction	

Table 3. Primary and secondary prevention statin trials.

The most important side effects associated with statins are hepatic injury and myopathy [64, 65]. The risk of liver injury with the use of statins appears to be dose dependent and is most likely to occur in the first 3 months. This risk was demonstrated in a meta-analysis of 35 randomized trials that showed an excess risk of 4.2 cases per 1000 patients associated with statin use [66]. Multiple mechanisms of liver injury have been demonstrated with statins including hepatocellular and cholestatic [67]. Among the different statins, the risk of liver injury appears to be similar, except with fluvastatin that has a higher risk [68]. Numerous studies have found no significant difference in elevated aminotransferases when statins were compared to placebo [25, 28, 57]. It was for this reason that the Food and Drug Administration

(FDA) revised the recommendation for liver function testing with regard to statin therapy in 2012 [69]. In the setting of rising aminotransferases three times the upper limit of normal, it is recommended to lower the statin dose or change medication.

Statin muscle injury remains the most concerning side effect, despite severe myopathy occurring in only 0.1–0.5% of patients [70, 71]. The degree of injury ranges from myalgia, myopathy, myositis, myonecrosis, to rhabdomyolysis [65]. Rhabdomyolysis, the most severe of the statin myopathy spectrum, was largely seen when statins were used with gemfibrozil or cyclosporine [72, 73]. This is thought to be related to the decrease in mevalonic acid associated with HMG-CoA reductase inhibition. Other mechanisms attributed to muscle injury include statins' effects on coenzyme Q10, also called ubiquinone, which is involved in muscle energy production [74]. Different statins possess varying risk to cause muscle injury, with fluvastatin exhibiting the lowest risk and simvastatin exhibiting a higher risk of muscle injury, especially at 80 mg/day dose, as shown in the SEARCH trial that was the basis of the FDA restriction of this dose of simvastatin [64, 70, 75]. The major predisposing factor for statin-induced myopathy injury includes hypothyroidism, obstructive liver disease, and renal failure; these contribute to both hypercholesterolemia and myopathy. Thus, it is important to test for thyroid-stimulating hormone (TSH) levels prior to starting statins [76].

Other notable side effects include proteinuria that has been reported to the Food and Drug Administration with rosuvastatin and simvastatin, but no increased risk of renal failure has been described [77–79]. In addition, there have been several meta-analyses of randomized trials that found a small, yet increased risk of diabetes with high-dose statin therapy when compared to lower-dose statin therapies, possibly related directly to its inhibition of HMG-CoA reductase [80]. However, given that statins have been shown to reduce CV events in diabetics, these studies have suggested that the beneficial effects of statins on CV events outweigh this risk [80, 81].

Despite physicians in practice witnessing the discontinuation of statins due to "intolerance," randomized control trials have failed to validate this finding. The difference between clinical practice and trials may relate to selection bias observed in clinical trials that limit their external validity [66, 82]. Intolerance is largely seen on the basis of muscle pain, leading to discontinuation of therapy. Another cause of intolerance is a rise in aminotransferases, which usually requires statins dose reduction, switch to another statin, or using an alternate drug. In patients, who are unable to tolerate statins, ezetimibe, fenofibrate, cholestyramine, and niacin have been recommended for those with known coronary heart disease (CHD) or at high-risk CV events (10-year risk >20%) [33]. Another option is the recently FDA-approved proprotein convertase subtilisin kexin type 9 (PCSK9) inhibitors.

2.2. PCSK9 inhibitors

PCSK9 is a serine protease that is mainly secreted by the liver in an inactive form, before undergoing catalytic changes in the endoplasmic reticulum. The mature PCSK9 is then released into the plasma where it has only one substrate, LDL receptors. Once in circulation, it regulates the LDL receptor recycling in the liver, intestines, pancreas, lungs, kidneys, and adipose tissue [83, 84]. PCSK9 binding to LDL receptors causes it to be internalized into endosomal or lysosomal compartments, where they are destroyed. This leads to a decrease in LDL receptors on the surface of the cell. It has therefore been shown that serum PCSK9 levels are inversely proportional to the number of LDL receptors (see **Figure 3**) [85, 86]. Blood levels of PCSK9 are influenced by the diurnal trend in secretion (peak levels at 4 am), gender (higher in females), and fasting states (lower levels) [87, 88]. A mutation in PCSK9 was first described in French families in 2003. It is the third gene implicated in the autosomal dominant familial hypercholesterolemia (FH); the other two genes encode LDL receptor and Apo-B, a component of the LDL particle [89]. It is usually a gain-of-function mutation in PCSK9 that results in a low level of LDL receptors leading to a high level of LDL and consequently increased risk of premature CV disease [90, 91]. On the other hand, loss-of-function PCSK9 mutations result in high level of LDL receptors, and a decrease in LDL and significant reduction in CV events. Of note, the reduction of CV events observed with PCSK9 mutation is higher than that associated with statins. This difference is attributed to the persistently low LDL levels caused by the underlying genetic predisposition. This was demonstrated in the ARIC study, Copenhagen Heart Study, and the Zimbabwe population study [92–94].

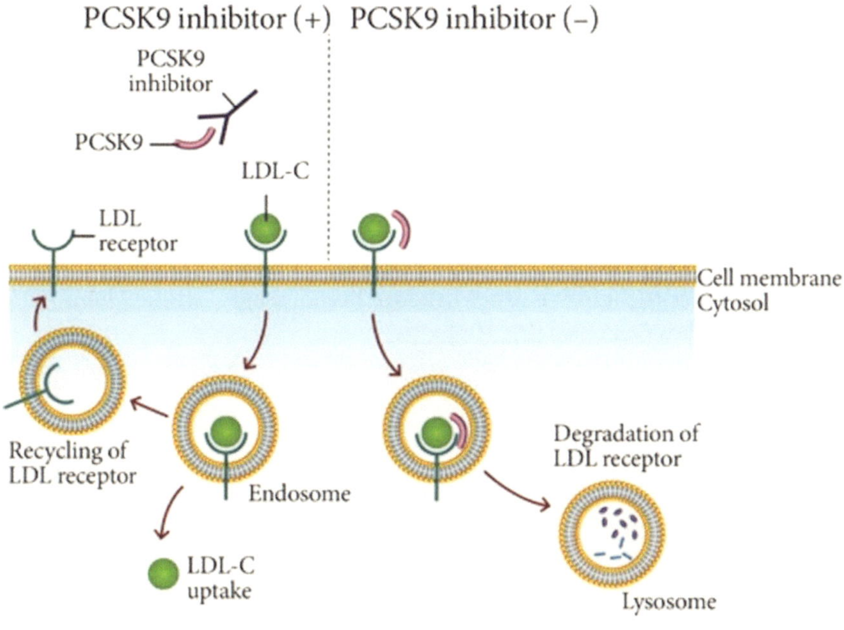

Figure 3. Mechanisms of PCSK9 inhibitors. Secreted PCSK9 binds to LDL receptors on the cell surface and forms an endosome that undergoes lysosomal degradation. In the presence of PCSK9 inhibitors, the interaction between PCSK9 and LDL receptors is disrupted, resulting in the recycling of LDL receptors and increased hepatic uptake of LDL from the bloodstream. *Abbreviations*: LDL, low-density lipoprotein cholesterol; PCSK9, proprotein convertase subtilisin kexin 9.

Statins have been described to increase the concentration of PCSK9 inhibitors by 14–47% in a dose- and time-dependent fashion. This is via a decrease in endogenous cholesterol synthesis caused by statin inhibition of HMG-CoA reductase with consequent up-regulation in LDL receptors. It has therefore been demonstrated that a PCSK9 mutation increases the response to statins [95–98]. Neutralizing antibodies to PCSK9 were first described in 2009, and in subsequent studies it was shown to decrease LDL levels by 30% in animal models [99].

Although statins are the most effective cholesterol-lowering agents for preventing CV events, there is a need for additional therapies in those patients who are (1) unable to take statins or (2) already on maximal statin doses with residual CV risk. The National Lipid Association in the US estimates that about 12% of patients discontinue statin therapy, of whom 62% experienced adverse effects [100]. These data signal the need for alternative effective agents, such as PCSK9 inhibitors, to be used with or instead of statins. As monotherapy, PCSK9 inhibitors lower LDL by up to approximately 66% [101]. In conjunction with statins, PCSK9 inhibitors reduce LDL by an additional 60% beyond statins [102]. Examples of monoclonal antibody PCSK9 inhibitors available in the market include evolocumab and alirocumab. Phase I, II, and III clinical trials have shown an additional decrease in LDL levels with the use of PCSK-9 inhibitors (monoclonal antibodies) in combination with statin therapy, as well as a significant decrease in CV events including mortality (hazard ratio (HR): 0.47–0.52) [2, 3]. Other PCSK9 inhibitors include the small interfering RNA (siRNA) molecules that block the synthesis of PCSK9 inhibitors and have been shown to decrease LDL by 40% in a phase I clinical trial when used at the highest dose compared to placebo [103].

Regarding their side effects, there were no significant differences in the incidence of adverse drug events between PCSK9 inhibitors (alirocumab, evolocumab) and placebo in the latest phase III trials, except for neurocognitive events, myalgia, injection site reactions, and ophthalmologic events [2, 3]. A major concern with PCSK9 inhibitors revolves around their cost and the very low LDL levels achieved (as low as 18 mg/dL compared to 44 mg/dL with rosuvastatin in the JUPITER study). Potential short- and long-term consequences of very low LDL levels include neurocognitive impairment, hemorrhagic stroke, hemolytic anemia, vitamin, and hormonal deficiencies [21, 104].

2.3. Ezetimibe

Ezetimibe inhibits the intestinal absorption of dietary and biliary cholesterol without affecting the absorption of fat-soluble vitamins or TG [105]. This possibly occurs by the inhibition of Niemann-Pick C1-like 1 (NPC1L1) protein function that is expressed in the intestines and liver [106]. The benefits of ezetimibe were demonstrated in the IMPROVE-IT trial where the addition of ezetimibe to statin therapy led to a decrease in CV events, excluding all-cause and CV mortality [54]. Ezetimibe is helpful in avoiding high doses of statin and the associated dose-dependent statin side effects, especially in patients who do not meet cholesterol targets. It has been well tolerated with the incidence of myopathy and serum transaminase elevations being similar when compared to placebo [54].

2.4. Bile acid sequestrants

Bile acid sequestrants, such as cholestyramine, colesevelam, and colestipol, lower cholesterol by binding to bile acids in the intestine preventing them from being reabsorbed [107]. The consequent decrease in intrahepatic cholesterol leads to an increase in LDL receptors that bind LDL from plasma with consequent small increase in HDL via increased intestinal synthesis of HDL [108]. They are relatively potent and exhibit a dose-dependent response achieving 10–25% reduction in LDL, exhibiting a synergistic effect when used with statins or niacin [55, 109, 110].

Major side effects have limited its overall use. Those described include abdominal discomfort with nausea, bloating, cramping, and rise in aminotransferases. Of the bile acid sequestrants, colesevelam is the better-tolerated drug. They also interact with common CV medications (warfarin and digoxin) by binding and inhibiting their absorption. This can be avoided by administering the other medications 1 h before or 4 h after ingestion of bile acid sequestrants [107].

2.5. Fibrates

Fibrates include gemfibrozil and fenofibrate [111]. The mechanism of action of fibrates is via activation of transcription factor, peroxisome proliferator-activated receptors (PPARs). It decreases TG via reduction in hepatic VLDL secretion, and stimulation of lipoprotein lipase that consequently leads to increased clearance of TG-rich lipoproteins. It also raises HDL by direct stimulation of HDL Apolipoprotein A-I/A-II synthesis and increased transfer of Apo A-I from HDL to VLDL [112].

This class of drugs lowers serum TG by 35–50%, and have also been shown to increase HDL by 5–20% directly proportional to the degree of hypertriglyceridemia [113–115]. Fibrates have not demonstrated any significant effect on cardiovascular outcomes, as seen in the FIELD trial [115], except in those with high TG (>200 mg/dL) or low HDL (<40 mg/dL) and metabolic syndrome, as was seen in the BIP trial [116].

The main side effect associated with fibrates is muscle injury. Muscle injury is often seen in patients who are already on a statin, and is thought to be mediated by fibrate-related inhibition of CYP3A4 with consequent decrease in statin metabolism [117]. Fibrates have also been shown to raise serum creatinine levels, but it remains unknown if there is direct parenchymal or tubular renal injury. Nevertheless, elevated creatinine has been found to be reversible on discontinuation of the medication, as was demonstrated in the FIELD trial [118]. Another noteworthy side effect is pancreatitis, which has been seen in patients with normal TG. However, the absolute risk remains low (number needed to harm over 5 years = 935) [119].

2.6. Nicotinic acid (niacin)

Nicotinic acid acts by inhibiting the hepatic production of VLDL and consequently decreasing LDL. It also increases HDL by reducing lipid transfer from HDL to VLDL, thus delaying HDL clearance [120]. This class of drugs has positive effects on HDL that occurs at relatively low dosages (1–1.5 g/day result in about 33% increase in HDL). Higher nicotinic acid doses are needed to lower LDL (3 g/day results in about 23% LDL decrease) [121, 122]. This class of drugs is also associated with a significant reduction of MACE in the HATS trial and ARBITER 6-HALTS trial when niacin was added to statin therapy [123, 124]. Contrary to these studies, the

AIM-HIGH, ARBITER-2, and HPS2-THRIVE trials found no significant benefit of adding niacin to statin therapy [125–127].

Unfortunately, its use is limited by poor tolerability. The most common side effect is flushing, which occurs in the majority (up to 80%) of patients at standard recommended doses. Other notable side effects include paresthesia, pruritis, and nausea, each of which occurs in 20% of patients at standard doses [120].

3. Lifestyle modification

All patients with an elevated LDL should be advised to attempt and undergo for therapeutic lifestyle changes. Therapeutic lifestyle changes involve weight loss (even in those who are only slightly overweight), exercise, and improvement in diet. Numerous studies have investigated and demonstrated the benefits of lifestyle modification. In the United Kingdom Lipid Clinics Program study, 2508 subjects who underwent diet modification experienced a 5–7% reduction in serum total and LDL cholesterol [128]. In the Lifestyle Heart Trial, 53 patients were randomized to either control diet (National Cholesterol Education Program-NCEP step 2 diet) or vegetarian therapy with exercise and relaxation therapy (intervention group). After 5 years of follow-up, the intervention group demonstrated a decrease in CV events (0.89 vs 2.25 events per patient) [129]. In the Lyon Diet Heart Study, 605 patients were randomized after a first myocardial infarction to either a Mediterranean diet or a control diet. After 4 years of follow-up, the Mediterranean diet group demonstrated lower rates of death and myocardial infarction [130].

4. Other potential therapy options

Statins are the preferred therapy for most patients with dyslipidemia, especially those with elevated total cholesterol and LDL cholesterol. However, in patients on maximal tolerated statin dose with a persistently elevated LDL, other therapies may be considered. These include niacin, bile acid sequestrants, and ezetimibe. Not uncommonly, these additional agents may not be sufficient to "normalize" abnormal cholesterol profiles, especially in patients with severe hypercholesterolemia and familial cholesterol diseases. Therapeutic options in this group of patients, who remain "at risk" for CV events, include LDL apheresis, lomitapide, surgical options, and gene therapy. Preferably, this cohort of patients should be managed by a specialist.

4.1. LDL apheresis

LDL apheresis is a procedure that involves extracorporeal removal of circulating Apo B-containing lipoprotein (e.g., LDL, VLDL, and lipoprotein-a). Regimens include weekly or biweekly depending on the rate LDL returns to baseline after therapy [131].

The National Lipid Associated Expert Panel on familial hypercholesterolemia recommended LDL apheresis in those with FH if LDL targets are not achieved with maximal tolerated medical therapy. These targets include LDL of ≥300 mg/dL in those with functional homozygous or heterozygous FH, LDL of ≥200 mg/dL in those with functional heterozygous FH, and ≥2 risk factors or high lipoprotein-a (≥50 mg/dL), or LDL of ≥160 mg/dL in those established CAD, CV disease, or diabetes [132]. In the absence of statin therapy, LDL apheresis lowers LDL by 50–75% acutely, by 30% after 6 months, and 38% after 18 months [133]. There are numerous studies showing benefit in outcomes such as myocardial infarction and reduction in arterial inflammation, but none have shown a survival benefit [134, 135]. Limitations to using LDL apheresis include patient burden, problems related to venous access, frequent long visits, and high costs [136].

4.2. Lomitapide

Lomitapide is a microsomal TG transfer protein inhibitor which inhibits the transfer of TG to Apo-B for the production of VLDL in the liver. However, lomitapide is metabolized by CYP3A4 and is also an inhibitor of CYP 3A4 and P-glycoprotein leading to numerous drug interactions. It was FDA approved in 2012 for use in patients with homozygous FH. It is used in addition to standard therapy, as well as other therapies such as LDL apheresis or liver transplantation. It has been shown to significantly decrease LDL (up to 50%) in a phase 3, open-label, non-randomized, dose-escalating study [137].

4.3. Mipomersen

Mipomersen is an injected antisense oligonucleotide that inhibits the production of Apo-B. Mipomersen binds to the Apo-B mRNA, affects Apo-B production, and consequently reduces the levels of LDL, VLDL, and intermediate dense lipoprotein. It has been approved by FDA in 2013 for use in homozygous FH patients; however, it is not approved in Europe. It has been shown that mipomersen can significantly decrease LDL in those patients with homozygous FH (up to 25%) [138]. Similar findings were found in studies involving other populations, including those with heterozygous FH and have CAD, statin intolerant, and at high risk of CV disease, and in those without FH who have or are at high risk of CVD [139–143].

4.4. Cholesteryl ester transfer protein inhibitors

Cholesteryl ester transfer protein (CETP) inhibitors, such as anacetrapib, have shown to significantly increase in HDL and lower LDL; however, there are no studies showing clinical benefit. In fact, in the REALIZE trial, despite a significant reduction in LDL in the intervention group compared to placebo, there was a significant increase in CV events, hence limiting its clinical use [144].

4.5. Anti-resistin antibodies

Anti-resistin antibodies inhibit resistin function, an adipokine (protein derived from adipose tissue) that is increased in obese individuals and positively correlated with atherosclerosis. In *in vitro* studies, resistin can decrease LDL receptor expression and increase PCSK9 expression.

By using anti-resistin antibodies, studies have shown an increase in LDL receptors in obese individuals [145].

4.6. Small molecule regulator of lipid metabolism

ETC-1002 is a small molecule regulator of carbohydrate and lipid metabolism. In a study of 177 subjects with LDL between 130 and 220 mg/dL not on statin therapy, patients were randomized to ETC-1002 (one of three different doses) or placebo. After 12 weeks of follow-up, treated subjects at the highest dose demonstrated a 27% decrease in LDL. There were no changes in TG or HDL. ETC-1002 also demonstrated a limited side effect profile [146, 147].

4.7. Recombinant Apo-A-I milano

Apo-A-I milano is a variant of the Apolipoprotein A-I (Apo-A-I). This variant leads to rapid mobilization of cholesterol with rapid regression of atherosclerosis. Subjects with Apo-A-I Milano have very low levels of HDL (10–30 mg/dL), longer survival, and reduced atherosclerosis compared to what is expected for their HDL levels [148]. Infusion of recombinant Apo-A-I milano (ETC-216) in an RCT was shown to lead to a significant regression of coronary atherosclerosis [149].

4.8. Lipoprotein-associated phospholipase A_2

Lipoprotein-associated phospholipase A_2 is also known as platelet-activating factor acetylhydrolase. It is a protein with pro-inflammatory properties that co-travels with circulating LDL particles and is found abundantly in atherosclerotic plaques [150]. Lipoprotein-associated phospholipase A_2 has been shown in a meta-analysis to significantly increase CHD and is an independent predictor of CHD and ischemic stroke [151]. However, in a large phase III randomized control trial (STABILITY trial), the lipoprotein-associated phospholipase A_2 inhibitor, darapladib, failed to show any CV benefit [152].

5. Conclusion

Over the last several years, the role of cholesterol-lowering agents in reducing cardiovascular disease and mortality has been further established. Statin therapy remains the cornerstone of lipid-lowering therapy; however, in patients already on maximal dose of statins or intolerant to statins with residual CV risk, other options are also available. As evidenced by the recent bench to bedside development of a new drug class (PCSK9), the emergence of drugs to specifically target a population, in this case, familial hypercholesterolemia, the national call for precision medicine is on the horizon. By continuing to scientifically probe biologic mechanisms in preclinical models related to cholesterol perturbation, drug development and translation to human clinical studies marks a bright and promising future.

http://dx.doi.org/10.5772/64762

Conflicts of interest

None.

Author details

Zaid Almarzooq and Parmanand Singh*

*Address all correspondence to: pas9062@med.cornell.edu

Weill Cornell Medical College, New York Presbyterian Hospital, New York, NY, USA

References

[1] Go AS, Mozaffarian D, Roger VL, Benjamin EJ, Berry JD, Borden WB, et al. Heart disease and stroke statistics—2013 update: a report from the American Heart Association. Circulation. 2013;127(1):e6.

[2] Sabatine MS, Giugliano RP, Wiviott SD, Raal FJ, Blom DJ, Robinson J, et al. Efficacy and safety of evolocumab in reducing lipids and cardiovascular events. N Engl J Med. 2015;372(16):1500–9.

[3] Robinson JG, Farnier M, Krempf M, Bergeron J, Luc G, Averna M, et al. Efficacy and safety of alirocumab in reducing lipids and cardiovascular events. N Engl J Med. 2015;372(16):1489–99.

[4] Expert Panel on Detection E. Executive summary of the Third Report of the National Cholesterol Education Program (NCEP) expert panel on detection, evaluation, and treatment of high blood cholesterol in adults (Adult Treatment Panel III). JAMA. 2001;285(19):2486.

[5] Salonen R, Nyyssönen K, Porkkala-Sarataho E, Salonen JT. The Kuopio Atherosclerosis Prevention Study (KAPS): effect of pravastatin treatment on lipids, oxidation resistance of lipoproteins, and atherosclerotic progression. Am J Cardiol. 1995;76(9):34C–9C.

[6] Jukema JW, Bruschke AV, van Boven AJ, Reiber JH, Bal ET, Zwinderman AH, et al. Effects of lipid lowering by pravastatin on progression and regression of coronary artery disease in symptomatic men with normal to moderately elevated serum cholesterol levels. The Regression Growth Evaluation Statin Study (REGRESS). Circulation. 1995;91(10):2528–40.

[7] Schartl M, Bocksch W, Koschyk DH, Voelker W, Karsch KR, Kreuzer J, et al. Use of intravascular ultrasound to compare effects of different strategies of lipid-lowering

therapy on plaque volume and composition in patients with coronary artery disease. Circulation. 2001;104(4):387–92.

[8] Nissen SE, Tuzcu EM, Schoenhagen P, Brown BG, Ganz P, Vogel RA, et al. Effect of intensive compared with moderate lipid-lowering therapy on progression of coronary atherosclerosis: a randomized controlled trial. JAMA. 2004;291(9):1071–80.

[9] Lee JM, Robson MD, Yu LM, Shirodaria CC, Cunnington C, Kylintireas I, et al. Effects of high-dose modified-release nicotinic acid on atherosclerosis and vascular function: a randomized, placebo-controlled, magnetic resonance imaging study. J Am Coll Cardiol. 2009;54(19):1787–94.

[10] Mihaylova B, Emberson J, Blackwell L, Keech A, Simes J, Barnes EH, et al. The effects of lowering LDL cholesterol with statin therapy in people at low risk of vascular disease: meta-analysis of individual data from 27 randomised trials. Lancet. 2012;380(9841):581–90.

[11] Genest J. Lipoprotein disorders and cardiovascular risk. J Inherit Metab Dis. 2003;26(2–3):267–87.

[12] Goldstein JL, Brown MS. The LDL receptor. Arterioscler Thromb Vasc Biol. 2009;29(4):431–8.

[13] Pekkanen J, Linn S, Heiss G, Suchindran CM, Leon A, Rifkind BM, et al. Ten-year mortality from cardiovascular disease in relation to cholesterol level among men with and without preexisting cardiovascular disease. N Engl J Med. 1990;322(24):1700–7.

[14] Collaboration PS. Blood cholesterol and vascular mortality by age, sex, and blood pressure: a meta-analysis of individual data from 61 prospective studies with 55 000 vascular deaths. Lancet. 2007;370(9602):1829–39.

[15] Pencina MJ, Navar-Boggan AM, D'Agostino RB, Sr., Williams K, Neely B, Sniderman AD, et al. Application of new cholesterol guidelines to a population-based sample. N Engl J Med. 2014;370(15):1422–31.

[16] Panel NCEPNE. Third Report of the National Cholesterol Education Program (NCEP) Expert Panel on Detection, Evaluation, and Treatment of High Blood Cholesterol in Adults (Adult Treatment Panel III) final report. Circulation. 2002;106(25):3143.

[17] Hayward RA, Krumholz HM. Three reasons to abandon low-density lipoprotein targets: an open letter to the Adult Treatment Panel IV of the National Institutes of Health. Circ Cardiovasc Qual Outcomes. 2012;5(1):2–5.

[18] Ray KK, Kastelein JJ, Boekholdt SM, Nicholls SJ, Khaw KT, Ballantyne CM, et al. The ACC/AHA 2013 guideline on the treatment of blood cholesterol to reduce atherosclerotic cardiovascular disease risk in adults: the good the bad and the uncertain: a comparison with ESC/EAS guidelines for the management of dyslipidaemias 2011. Eur Heart J. 2014;35(15):960–8.

[19] Bu DX, Griffin G, Lichtman AH. Mechanisms for the anti-inflammatory effects of statins. Curr Opin Lipidol. 2011;22(3):165–70.

[20] Glynn RJ, Koenig W, Nordestgaard BG, Shepherd J, Ridker PM. Rosuvastatin for primary prevention in older persons with elevated C-reactive protein and low to average low-density lipoprotein cholesterol levels: exploratory analysis of a randomized trial. Ann Intern Med. 2010;152(8):488–96, W174.

[21] Hsia J, MacFadyen JG, Monyak J, Ridker PM. Cardiovascular event reduction and adverse events among subjects attaining low-density lipoprotein cholesterol< 50 mg/dl with rosuvastatin: the JUPITER trial (Justification for the Use of Statins in Prevention: an Intervention Trial Evaluating Rosuvastatin). J Am Coll Cardiol. 2011;57(16):1666–75.

[22] Nissen SE, Tuzcu EM, Schoenhagen P, Crowe T, Sasiela WJ, Tsai J, et al. Statin therapy, LDL cholesterol, C-reactive protein, and coronary artery disease. N Engl J Med. 2005;352(1):29–38.

[23] Puri R, Nissen SE, Libby P, Shao M, Ballantyne CM, Barter PJ, et al. C-reactive protein, but not low-density lipoprotein cholesterol levels, associate with coronary atheroma regression and cardiovascular events following maximally intensive statin therapy. Circulation. 2013:CIRCULATIONAHA. 113.004243.

[24] Varbo A, Benn M, Tybjaerg-Hansen A, Nordestgaard BG. Elevated remnant cholesterol causes both low-grade inflammation and ischemic heart disease, whereas elevated low-density lipoprotein cholesterol causes ischemic heart disease without inflammation. Circulation. 2013;128(12):1298–309.

[25] Collins R, Armitage J, Parish S, Sleight P, Peto R, Collaboration HPS. MRC/BHF Heart Protection Study of cholesterol lowering with simvastatin in 20 536 high-risk individuals: a randomised placebo controlled trial. Lancet. 2002;360(9326):7–22.

[26] Colhoun HM, Betteridge DJ, Durrington PN, Hitman GA, Neil HA, Livingstone SJ, et al. Primary prevention of cardiovascular disease with atorvastatin in type 2 diabetes in the Collaborative Atorvastatin Diabetes Study (CARDS): multicentre randomised placebo-controlled trial. Lancet. 2004;364(9435):685–96.

[27] Nakamura H, Arakawa K, Itakura H, Kitabatake A, Goto Y, Toyota T, et al. Primary prevention of cardiovascular disease with pravastatin in Japan (MEGA Study): a prospective randomised controlled trial. Lancet. 2006;368(9542):1155–63.

[28] Group SSSS. Randomised trial of cholesterol lowering in 4444 patients with coronary heart disease: the Scandinavian Simvastatin Survival Study (4S). Lancet. 1994;344(8934):1383–9.

[29] Marschner IC, Colquhoun D, Simes RJ, Glasziou P, Harris P, Singh BB, et al. Long-term risk stratification for survivors of acute coronary syndromes. Results from the Long-term Intervention with Pravastatin in Ischemic Disease (LIPID) Study. LIPID Study Investigators. J Am Coll Cardiol. 2001;38(1):56–63.

[30] Schwartz GG, Olsson AG, Ezekowitz MD, Ganz P, Oliver MF, Waters D, et al. Effects of atorvastatin on early recurrent ischemic events in acute coronary syndromes: the MIRACL study: a randomized controlled trial. JAMA. 2001;285(13):1711–8.

[31] LaRosa JC, He J, Vupputuri S. Effect of statins on risk of coronary disease: a meta-analysis of randomized controlled trials. JAMA. 1999;282(24):2340–6.

[32] Cannon CP, Braunwald E, McCabe CH, Rader DJ, Rouleau JL, Belder R, et al. Intensive versus moderate lipid lowering with statins after acute coronary syndromes. N Engl J Med. 2004;350(15):1495–504.

[33] Navarese EP, Kolodziejczak M, Schulze V, Gurbel PA, Tantry U, Lin Y, et al. Effects of proprotein convertase subtilisin/kexin type 9 antibodies in adults with hypercholesterolemia: a systematic review and meta-analysis. Ann Intern Med. 2015;163(1):40–51.

[34] D'Agostino RB, Vasan RS, Pencina MJ, Wolf PA, Cobain M, Massaro JM, et al. General cardiovascular risk profile for use in primary care the Framingham Heart Study. Circulation. 2008;117(6):743–53.

[35] Muntner P, Colantonio LD, Cushman M, Goff DC, Jr., Howard G, Howard VJ, et al. Validation of the atherosclerotic cardiovascular disease pooled cohort risk equations. JAMA. 2014;311(14):1406–15.

[36] Board JBS. Joint British Societies' consensus recommendations for the prevention of cardiovascular disease (JBS3). Heart. 2014;100(Suppl 2):ii1–67.

[37] Stevens RJ, Kothari V, Adler AI, Stratton IM, United Kingdom Prospective Diabetes Study G. The UKPDS risk engine: a model for the risk of coronary heart disease in type II diabetes (UKPDS 56). Clin Sci (Lond). 2001;101(6):671–9.

[38] Pandya A, Sy S, Cho S, Weinstein MC, Gaziano TA. Cost-effectiveness of 10-year risk thresholds for initiation of statin therapy for primary prevention of cardiovascular disease. JAMA. 2015;314(2):142–50.

[39] Grundy SM, Cleeman JI, Rifkind BM, Kuller LH. Cholesterol lowering in the elderly population. Coordinating Committee of the National Cholesterol Education Program. Arch Intern Med. 1999;159(15):1670–8.

[40] Miettinen TA, Pyorala K, Olsson AG, Musliner TA, Cook TJ, Faergeman O, et al. Cholesterol-lowering therapy in women and elderly patients with myocardial infarction or angina pectoris: findings from the Scandinavian Simvastatin Survival Study (4S). Circulation. 1997;96(12):4211–8.

[41] LaRosa JC, Grundy SM, Waters DD, Shear C, Barter P, Fruchart JC, et al. Intensive lipid lowering with atorvastatin in patients with stable coronary disease. N Engl J Med. 2005;352(14):1425–35.

[42] Istvan ES, Deisenhofer J. Structural mechanism for statin inhibition of HMG-CoA reductase. Science. 2001;292(5519):1160–4.

[43] Haslinger-Löffler B. Multiple effects of HMG-CoA reductase inhibitors (statins) besides their lipid-lowering function. Kidney Int. 2008;74(5):553–5.

[44] Ness GC, Zhao Z, Lopez D. Inhibitors of cholesterol biosynthesis increase hepatic low-density lipoprotein receptor protein degradation. Arch Biochem Biophys. 1996;325(2): 242–8.

[45] Ness GC, Chambers CM, Lopez D. Atorvastatin action involves diminished recovery of hepatic HMG-CoA reductase activity. J Lipid Res. 1998;39(1):75–84.

[46] Arad Y, Ramakrishnan R, Ginsberg HN. Lovastatin therapy reduces low density lipoprotein ApoB levels in subjects with combined hyperlipidemia by reducing the production of ApoB-containing lipoproteins: implications for the pathophysiology of ApoB production. J Lipid Res. 1990;31(4):567–82.

[47] Niesor EJ, Schwartz GG, Perez A, Stauffer A, Durrwell A, Bucklar-Suchankova G, et al. Statin-induced decrease in ATP-binding cassette transporter A1 expression via microRNA33 induction may counteract cholesterol efflux to high-density lipoprotein. Cardiovasc Drugs Ther. 2015;29(1):7–14.

[48] Davignon J, Ganz P. Role of endothelial dysfunction in atherosclerosis. Circulation. 2004;109(23 Suppl 1):III27–32.

[49] Rosenson RS, Otvos JD, Hsia J. Effects of rosuvastatin and atorvastatin on LDL and HDL particle concentrations in patients with metabolic syndrome: a randomized, double-blind, controlled study. Diabetes Care. 2009;32(6):1087–91.

[50] Otvos JD, Shalaurova I, Freedman DS, Rosenson RS. Effects of pravastatin treatment on lipoprotein subclass profiles and particle size in the PLAC-I trial. Atherosclerosis. 2002;160(1):41–8.

[51] Jones PH, Davidson MH, Stein EA, Bays HE, McKenney JM, Miller E, et al. Comparison of the efficacy and safety of rosuvastatin versus atorvastatin, simvastatin, and pravastatin across doses (STELLAR* Trial). Am J Cardiol. 2003;92(2):152–60.

[52] Jones P, Kafonek S, Laurora I, Hunninghake D. Comparative dose efficacy study of atorvastatin versus simvastatin, pravastatin, lovastatin, and fluvastatin in patients with hypercholesterolemia (the CURVES study). Am J Cardiol. 1998;81(5): 582–7.

[53] Stender S, Budinski D, Gosho M, Hounslow N. Pitavastatin shows greater lipid-lowering efficacy over 12 weeks than pravastatin in elderly patients with primary hypercholesterolaemia or combined (mixed) dyslipidaemia. Eur J Preventive Cardiol. 2013;20(1):40–53.

[54] Cannon CP, Blazing MA, Giugliano RP, McCagg A, White JA, Theroux P, et al. Ezetimibe added to statin therapy after acute coronary syndromes. N Engl J Med. 2015;372(25): 2387–97.

[55] Knopp RH, Brown WV, Corder CN, Dobs AS, Dujovne CA, Goldberg AC, et al. Comparative efficacy and safety of pravastatin and cholestyramine alone and combined in patients with hypercholesterolemia. Arch Int Med. 1993;153(11): 1321–9.

[56] Salonen R, Nyyssonen K, Porkkala E, Rummukainen J, Belder R, Park JS, et al. Kuopio Atherosclerosis Prevention Study (KAPS). A population-based primary preventive trial of the effect of LDL lowering on atherosclerotic progression in carotid and femoral arteries. Circulation. 1995;92(7):1758–64.

[57] Downs JR, Clearfield M, Weis S, Whitney E, Shapiro DR, Beere PA, et al. Primary prevention of acute coronary events with lovastatin in men and women with average cholesterol levels: results of AFCAPS/TexCAPS. Air Force/Texas Coronary Atherosclerosis Prevention Study. JAMA. 1998;279(20):1615–22.

[58] Pedersen TR, Faergeman O, Kastelein JJ, Olsson AG, Tikkanen MJ, Holme I, et al. High-dose atorvastatin vs usual-dose simvastatin for secondary prevention after myocardial infarction: the IDEAL study: a randomized controlled trial. JAMA. 2005;294(19):2437–45.

[59] Shepherd J, Blauw GJ, Murphy MB, Bollen ELEM, Buckley BM, Cobbe SM, et al. Pravastatin in elderly individuals at risk of vascular disease (PROSPER): a randomised controlled trial. Lancet. 2002;360(9346):1623–30.

[60] Group WS. Baseline characteristics and screening experience in the West of Scotland Coronary Prevention Study. Am J Cardiol. 1995;76:485–91.

[61] Furberg CD, Wright JT, Davis BR, Cutler JA, Alderman M, Black H, et al. Major outcomes in moderately hypercholesterolemic, hypertensive patients randomized to pravastatin vs usual care—the antihypertensive and lipid-lowering treatment to prevent heart attack trial (ALLHAT-LLT). JAMA—J Am Med Assoc. 2002;288(23):2998–3007.

[62] Lewis SJ, Moye LA, Sacks FM, Johnstone DE, Timmis G, Mitchell J, et al. Effect of pravastatin on cardiovascular events in older patients with myocardial infarction and cholesterol levels in the average range. Results of the Cholesterol and Recurrent Events (CARE) trial. Ann Intern Med. 1998;129(9):681–9.

[63] Group LS. Long-term effectiveness and safety of pravastatin in 9014 patients with coronary heart disease and average cholesterol concentrations: the LIPID trial follow-up. The Lancet. 2002;359(9315):1379–87.

[64] Stroes ES, Thompson PD, Corsini A, Vladutiu GD, Raal FJ, Ray KK, et al. Statin-associated muscle symptoms: impact on statin therapy-European Atherosclerosis Society Consensus Panel Statement on Assessment, Aetiology and Management. Eur Heart J. 2015;36(17):1012–22.

[65] Rosenson RS, Baker SK, Jacobson TA, Kopecky SL, Parker BA, The National Lipid Association's Muscle Safety Expert P. An assessment by the Statin Muscle Safety Task Force: 2014 update. J Clin Lipidol. 2014;8(3 Suppl):S58–71.

[66] Kashani A, Phillips CO, Foody JM, Wang Y, Mangalmurti S, Ko DT, et al. Risks associated with statin therapy: a systematic overview of randomized clinical trials. Circulation. 2006;114(25):2788–97.

[67] Russo MW, Hoofnagle JH, Gu J, Fontana RJ, Barnhart H, Kleiner DE, et al. Spectrum of statin hepatotoxicity: experience of the drug-induced liver injury network. Hepatology. 2014;60(2):679–86.

[68] Hippisley-Cox J, Coupland C. Unintended effects of statins in men and women in England and Wales: population based cohort study using the QResearch database. BMJ. 2010;340:c2197.

[69] Marcum ZA, Vande Griend JP, Linnebur SA. FDA drug safety communications: a narrative review and clinical considerations for older adults. Am J Geriatr Pharmacother. 2012;10(4):264–71.

[70] Graham DJ, Staffa JA, Shatin D, Andrade SE, Schech SD, La Grenade L, et al. Incidence of hospitalized rhabdomyolysis in patients treated with lipid-lowering drugs. JAMA. 2004;292(21):2585–90.

[71] Dujovne CA, Chremos AN, Pool JL, Schnaper H, Bradford RH, Shear CL, et al. Expanded clinical evaluation of lovastatin (EXCEL) study results: IV. Additional perspectives on the tolerability of lovastatin. Am J Med. 1991;91(1B):25S–30S.

[72] Norman DJ, Illingworth DR, Munson J, Hosenpud J. Myolysis and acute renal failure in a heart-transplant recipient receiving lovastatin. N Engl J Med. 1988;318(1):46–7.

[73] Pierce LR, Wysowski DK, Gross TP. Myopathy and rhabdomyolysis associated with lovastatin-gemfibrozil combination therapy. JAMA. 1990;264(1):71–5.

[74] Rundek T, Naini A, Sacco R, Coates K, DiMauro S. Atorvastatin decreases the coenzyme Q10 level in the blood of patients at risk for cardiovascular disease and stroke. Arch Neurol. 2004;61(6):889–92.

[75] Armitage J, Bowman L, Wallendszus K, Bulbulia R, Rahimi K, Haynes R, et al. Intensive lowering of LDL cholesterol with 80 mg versus 20 mg simvastatin daily in 12 064 survivors of myocardial infarction: a double-blind randomised trial. Lancet. 2010;376(9753):1658–69.

[76] Bar SL, Holmes DT, Frohlich J. Asymptomatic hypothyroidism and statin-induced myopathy. Can Fam Phys. 2007;53(3):428–31.

[77] Howard W. The issue of statin safety: where do we stand? Grundy SM (University of Texas Southwestern Med Ctr, Dallas) Circulation 111:301 (6–9), 2005. Year Book Endocrinol. 2006;2006:126–7.

[78] Jacobson TA. Statin safety: lessons from new drug applications for marketed statins. Am J Cardiol. 2006;97(8A):44C–51C.

[79] Alsheikh-Ali AA, Ambrose MS, Kuvin JT, Karas RH. The safety of rosuvastatin as used in common clinical practice: a postmarketing analysis. Circulation. 2005;111(23):3051–7.

[80] Swerdlow DI, Preiss D, Kuchenbaecker KB, Holmes MV, Engmann JE, Shah T, et al. HMG-coenzyme A reductase inhibition, type 2 diabetes, and bodyweight: evidence from genetic analysis and randomised trials. Lancet. 2015;385(9965):351–61.

[81] Preiss D, Seshasai SR, Welsh P, Murphy SA, Ho JE, Waters DD, et al. Risk of incident diabetes with intensive-dose compared with moderate-dose statin therapy: a meta-analysis. JAMA. 2011;305(24):2556–64.

[82] Armitage J. The safety of statins in clinical practice. Lancet. 2007;370(9601):1781–90.

[83] Benjannet S, Rhainds D, Essalmani R, Mayne J, Wickham L, Jin W, et al. NARC-1/PCSK9 and its natural mutants: zymogen cleavage and effects on the low density lipoprotein (LDL) receptor and LDL cholesterol. J Biol Chem. 2004;279(47):48865–75.

[84] Seidah NG, Benjannet S, Wickham L, Marcinkiewicz J, Jasmin SB, Stifani S, et al. The secretory proprotein convertase neural apoptosis-regulated convertase 1 (NARC-1): liver regeneration and neuronal differentiation. Proc Natl Acad Sci USA. 2003;100(3):928–33.

[85] Alborn WE, Cao G, Careskey HE, Qian YW, Subramaniam DR, Davies J, et al. Serum proprotein convertase subtilisin kexin type 9 is correlated directly with serum LDL cholesterol. Clin Chem. 2007;53(10):1814–9.

[86] Ahn CH, Choi SH. New drugs for treating dyslipidemia: beyond statins. Diabetes Metab J. 2015;39(2):87–94.

[87] Cui Q, Ju X, Yang T, Zhang M, Tang W, Chen Q, et al. Serum PCSK9 is associated with multiple metabolic factors in a large Han Chinese population. Atherosclerosis. 2010;213(2):632–6.

[88] Persson L, Cao G, Stahle L, Sjoberg BG, Troutt JS, Konrad RJ, et al. Circulating proprotein convertase subtilisin kexin type 9 has a diurnal rhythm synchronous with cholesterol synthesis and is reduced by fasting in humans. Arterioscler Thromb Vasc Biol. 2010;30(12):2666–72.

[89] Abifadel M, Varret M, Rabes JP, Allard D, Ouguerram K, Devillers M, et al. Mutations in PCSK9 cause autosomal dominant hypercholesterolemia. Nat Genet. 2003;34(2):154–6.

[90] Maxwell KN, Breslow JL. Proprotein convertase subtilisin kexin 9: the third locus implicated in autosomal dominant hypercholesterolemia. Curr Opin Lipidol. 2005;16(2):167–72.

[91] Humphries SE, Whittall RA, Hubbart CS, Maplebeck S, Cooper JA, Soutar AK, et al. Genetic causes of familial hypercholesterolaemia in patients in the UK: relation to plasma lipid levels and coronary heart disease risk. J Med Genet. 2006;43(12):943–9.

[92] Cohen JC, Boerwinkle E, Mosley TH, Jr., Hobbs HH. Sequence variations in PCSK9, low LDL, and protection against coronary heart disease. N Engl J Med. 2006;354(12):1264–72.

[93] Benn M, Nordestgaard BG, Grande P, Schnohr P, Tybjaerg-Hansen A. PCSK9 R46L, low-density lipoprotein cholesterol levels, and risk of ischemic heart disease: 3 independent studies and meta-analyses. J Am Coll Cardiol. 2010;55(25):2833–42.

[94] Hooper AJ, Marais AD, Tanyanyiwa DM, Burnett JR. The C679X mutation in PCSK9 is present and lowers blood cholesterol in a Southern African population. Atherosclerosis. 2007;193(2):445–8.

[95] Brown MS, Goldstein JL. A proteolytic pathway that controls the cholesterol content of membranes, cells, and blood. Proc Natl Acad Sci USA. 1999;96(20):11041–8.

[96] Dubuc G, Chamberland A, Wassef H, Davignon J, Seidah NG, Bernier L, et al. Statins upregulate PCSK9, the gene encoding the proprotein convertase neural apoptosis-regulated convertase-1 implicated in familial hypercholesterolemia. Arterioscler Thromb Vasc Biol. 2004;24(8):1454–9.

[97] Nohturfft A, DeBose-Boyd RA, Scheek S, Goldstein JL, Brown MS. Sterols regulate cycling of SREBP cleavage-activating protein (SCAP) between endoplasmic reticulum and Golgi. Proc Natl Acad Sci USA. 1999;96(20):11235–40.

[98] Berge KE, Ose L, Leren TP. Missense mutations in the PCSK9 gene are associated with hypocholesterolemia and possibly increased response to statin therapy. Arterioscler Thromb Vasc Biol. 2006;26(5):1094–100.

[99] Chan JC, Piper DE, Cao Q, Liu D, King C, Wang W, et al. A proprotein convertase subtilisin/kexin type 9 neutralizing antibody reduces serum cholesterol in mice and nonhuman primates. Proc Natl Acad Sci USA. 2009;106(24):9820–5.

[100] Toth PP, Harper CR, Jacobson TA. Clinical characterization and molecular mechanisms of statin myopathy. Expert Rev Cardiovasc Ther. 2008;6(7):955–69.

[101] Raal FJ, Stein EA, Dufour R, Turner T, Civeira F, Burgess L, et al. PCSK9 inhibition with evolocumab (AMG 145) in heterozygous familial hypercholesterolaemia (RUTHERFORD-2): a randomised, double-blind, placebo-controlled trial. Lancet. 2015;385(9965):331–40.

[102] Roth EM, McKenney JM, Hanotin C, Asset G, Stein EA. Atorvastatin with or without an antibody to PCSK9 in primary hypercholesterolemia. N Engl J Med. 2012;367(20):1891–900.

[103] Fitzgerald K, Frank-Kamenetsky M, Shulga-Morskaya S, Liebow A, Bettencourt BR, Sutherland JE, et al. Effect of an RNA interference drug on the synthesis of proprotein

convertase subtilisin/kexin type 9 (PCSK9) and the concentration of serum LDL cholesterol in healthy volunteers: a randomised, single-blind, placebo-controlled, phase 1 trial. Lancet. 2014;383(9911):60–8.

[104] LaRosa JC, Pedersen TR, Somaratne R, Wasserman SM. Safety and effect of very low levels of low-density lipoprotein cholesterol on cardiovascular events. Am J Cardiol. 2013;111(8):1221–9.

[105] Sudhop T, Lutjohann D, Kodal A, Igel M, Tribble DL, Shah S, et al. Inhibition of intestinal cholesterol absorption by ezetimibe in humans. Circulation. 2002;106(15):1943–8.

[106] Altmann SW, Davis HR, Jr., Zhu LJ, Yao X, Hoos LM, Tetzloff G, et al. Niemann-Pick C1 Like 1 protein is critical for intestinal cholesterol absorption. Science. 2004;303(5661): 1201–4.

[107] Davidson MH, Dillon MA, Gordon B, Jones P, Samuels J, Weiss S, et al. Colesevelam hydrochloride (cholestagel): a new, potent bile acid sequestrant associated with a low incidence of gastrointestinal side effects. Arch Intern Med. 1999;159(16):1893–900.

[108] Shepherd J, Packard CJ, Morgan HG, Third JL, Stewart JM, Lawrie TD. The effects of cholestyramine on high density lipoprotein metabolism. Atherosclerosis. 1979;33(4): 433–44.

[109] Insull W, Toth P, Mullican W, Hunninghake D, Burke S, Donovan JM, et al., editors. Effectiveness of colesevelam hydrochloride in decreasing LDL cholesterol in patients with primary hypercholesterolemia: a 24-week randomized controlled trial. Mayo Clinic Proceedings; 2001: Elsevier.

[110] Brown G, Albers JJ, Fisher LD, Schaefer SM, Lin JT, Kaplan C, et al. Regression of coronary artery disease as a result of intensive lipid-lowering therapy in men with high levels of Apolipoprotein B. N Engl J Med. 1990;323(19):1289–98.

[111] Oliver MF, Heady JA, Morris JN, Cooper MJ. Who cooperative trial on primary prevention of ischemic-heart-disease with clofibrate to lower serum-cholesterol—final mortality follow-up. Lancet. 1984;2(8403):600–4.

[112] Staels B, Dallongeville J, Auwerx J, Schoonjans K, Leitersdorf E, Fruchart JC. Mechanism of action of fibrates on lipid and lipoprotein metabolism. Circulation. 1998;98(19): 2088–93.

[113] Birjmohun RS, Hutten BA, Kastelein JJ, Stroes ES. Efficacy and safety of high-density lipoprotein cholesterol-increasing compounds: a meta-analysis of randomized controlled trials. J Am Coll Cardiol. 2005;45(2):185–97.

[114] Rubins HB, Robins SJ, Collins D, Fye CL, Anderson JW, Elam MB, et al. Gemfibrozil for the secondary prevention of coronary heart disease in men with low levels of high-density lipoprotein cholesterol. Veterans Affairs High-Density Lipoprotein Cholesterol Intervention Trial Study Group. N Engl J Med. 1999;341(6):410–8.

[115] Investigators FS. Effects of long-term fenofibrate therapy on cardiovascular events in 9795 people with type 2 diabetes mellitus (the FIELD study): randomised controlled trial. The Lancet. 2005;366(9500):1849–61.

[116] Group BS. Secondary prevention by raising HDL cholesterol and reducing triglycerides in patients with coronary artery disease the bezafibrate infarction prevention (BIP) study. Circulation. 2000;102(1):21–7.

[117] Athyros VG, Papageorgiou AA, Hatzikonstandinou HA, Didangelos TP, Carina MV, Kranitsas DF, et al. Safety and efficacy of long-term statin-fibrate combinations in patients with refractory familial combined hyperlipidemia. Am J Cardiol. 1997;80(5): 608–13.

[118] Davis TM, Ting R, Best JD, Donoghoe MW, Drury PL, Sullivan DR, et al. Effects of fenofibrate on renal function in patients with type 2 diabetes mellitus: the fenofibrate intervention and event lowering in diabetes (FIELD) study. Diabetologia. 2011;54(2): 280–90.

[119] Preiss D, Tikkanen MJ, Welsh P, Ford I, Lovato LC, Elam MB, et al. Lipid-modifying therapies and risk of pancreatitis: a meta-analysis. JAMA. 2012;308(8):804–11.

[120] Illingworth DR, Stein EA, Mitchel YB, Dujovne CA, Frost PH, Knopp RH, et al. Comparative effects of lovastatin and niacin in primary hypercholesterolemia. A prospective trial. Arch Intern Med. 1994;154(14):1586–95.

[121] Probstfield JL, Hunninghake DB. Nicotinic-acid as a lipoprotein-altering agent—therapy directed by the primary physician. Arch Int Med. 1994;154(14):1557–9.

[122] Grundy SM, Mok HY, Zech L, Berman M. Influence of nicotinic acid on metabolism of cholesterol and triglycerides in man. J Lipid Res. 1981;22(1):24–36.

[123] Zhao XQ, Morse JS, Dowdy AA, Heise N, DeAngelis D, Frohlich J, et al. Safety and tolerability of simvastatin plus niacin in patients with coronary artery disease and low high-density lipoprotein cholesterol (The HDL Atherosclerosis Treatment Study). Am J Cardiol. 2004;93(3):307–12.

[124] Villines TC, Stanek EJ, Devine PJ, Turco M, Miller M, Weissman NJ, et al. The ARBITER 6-HALTS Trial (arterial biology for the investigation of the treatment effects of reducing cholesterol 6-HDL and LDL treatment strategies in atherosclerosis): final results and the impact of medication adherence, dose, and treatment duration. J Am Coll Cardiol. 2010;55(24):2721–6.

[125] Investigators A-H, Boden WE, Probstfield JL, Anderson T, Chaitman BR, Desvignes-Nickens P, et al. Niacin in patients with low HDL cholesterol levels receiving intensive statin therapy. N Engl J Med. 2011;365(24):2255–67.

[126] Taylor AJ, Sullenberger LE, Lee HJ, Lee JK, Grace KA. Arterial biology for the investigation of the treatment effects of reducing cholesterol (ARBITER) 2: a double-blind,

placebo-controlled study of extended-release niacin on atherosclerosis progression in secondary prevention patients treated with statins. Circulation. 2004;110(23):3512–7.

[127] Group H-TC. Effects of extended-release niacin with laropiprant in high-risk patients. N Engl J Med. 2014;371(3):203.

[128] Butowski PF, Winder AF. Usual care dietary practice, achievement and implications for medication in the management of hypercholesterolaemia. Data from the U.K. Lipid Clinics Programme. Eur Heart J. 1998;19(9):1328–33.

[129] Ornish D, Scherwitz LW, Billings JH, Brown SE, Gould KL, Merritt TA, et al. Intensive lifestyle changes for reversal of coronary heart disease. JAMA. 1998;280(23):2001–7.

[130] Michel de Lorgeril M, Salen P, Martin J-L, Monjaud I, Delaye J, Mamelle N. Mediterranean diet, traditional risk factors, and the rate of cardiovascular complications after myocardial infarction. Heart Failure. 1999;11(6): 779–785.

[131] Thompson GR, Catapano A, Saheb S, Atassi-Dumont M, Barbir M, Eriksson M, et al. Severe hypercholesterolaemia: therapeutic goals and eligibility criteria for LDL apheresis in Europe. Curr Opin Lipidol. 2010;21(6):492–8.

[132] Ito MK, McGowan MP, Moriarty PM, National Lipid Association Expert Panel on Familial H. Management of familial hypercholesterolemias in adult patients: recommendations from the National Lipid Association Expert Panel on familial hypercholesterolemia. J Clin Lipidol. 2011;5(3 Suppl):S38–45.

[133] Hemphill LC. Familial hypercholesterolemia: current treatment options and patient selection for low-density lipoprotein apheresis. J Clin Lipidol. 2010;4(5):346–9.

[134] Mabuchi H, Koizumi J, Shimizu M, Kajinami K, Miyamoto S, Ueda K, et al. Long-term efficacy of low-density lipoprotein apheresis on coronary heart disease in familial hypercholesterolemia. Hokuriku-FH-LDL-Apheresis Study Group. Am J Cardiol. 1998;82(12):1489–95.

[135] van Wijk DF, Sjouke B, Figueroa A, Emami H, van der Valk FM, MacNabb MH, et al. Nonpharmacological lipoprotein apheresis reduces arterial inflammation in familial hypercholesterolemia. J Am Coll Cardiol. 2014;64(14):1418–26.

[136] Stefanutti C, Vivenzio A, Di Giacomo S, Mazzarella B, Bosco G, Berni A. Aorta and coronary angiographic follow-up of children with severe hypercholesterolemia treated with low-density lipoprotein apheresis. Transfusion. 2009;49(7):1461–70.

[137] Cuchel M, Meagher EA, du Toit Theron H, Blom DJ, Marais AD, Hegele RA, et al. Efficacy and safety of a microsomal triglyceride transfer protein inhibitor in patients with homozygous familial hypercholesterolaemia: a single-arm, open-label, phase 3 study. Lancet. 2013;381(9860):40–6.

[138] Raal FJ, Santos RD, Blom DJ, Marais AD, Charng MJ, Cromwell WC, et al. Mipomersen, an Apolipoprotein B synthesis inhibitor, for lowering of LDL cholesterol concentrations

in patients with homozygous familial hypercholesterolaemia: a randomised, double-blind, placebo-controlled trial. Lancet. 2010;375(9719):998–1006.

[139] Kastelein JJ, Wedel MK, Baker BF, Su J, Bradley JD, Yu RZ, et al. Potent reduction of Apolipoprotein B and low-density lipoprotein cholesterol by short-term administration of an antisense inhibitor of Apolipoprotein B. Circulation. 2006;114(16):1729–35.

[140] Akdim F, Stroes ES, Sijbrands EJ, Tribble DL, Trip MD, Jukema JW, et al. Efficacy and safety of mipomersen, an antisense inhibitor of Apolipoprotein B, in hypercholesterolemic subjects receiving stable statin therapy. J Am Coll Cardiol. 2010;55(15):1611–8.

[141] Stein EA, Dufour R, Gagne C, Gaudet D, East C, Donovan JM, et al. Apolipoprotein B synthesis inhibition with mipomersen in heterozygous familial hypercholesterolemia: results of a randomized, double-blind, placebo controlled trial to assess efficacy and safety as add-on therapy in patients with coronary artery disease. Circulation. 2012;126(19):2283–92. doi: 10.1161/CIRCULATIONAHA.112.104125.

[142] Visser ME, Wagener G, Baker BF, Geary RS, Donovan JM, Beuers UH, et al. Mipomersen, an Apolipoprotein B synthesis inhibitor, lowers low-density lipoprotein cholesterol in high-risk statin-intolerant patients: a randomized, double-blind, placebo-controlled trial. Eur Heart J. 2012;33(9):1142–9.

[143] Thomas GS, Cromwell WC, Ali S, Chin W, Flaim JD, Davidson M. Mipomersen, an Apolipoprotein B synthesis inhibitor, reduces atherogenic lipoproteins in patients with severe hypercholesterolemia at high cardiovascular risk: a randomized, double-blind, placebo-controlled trial. J Am Coll Cardiol. 2013;62(23):2178–84.

[144] Kastelein JJP, Besseling J, Shah S, Bergeron J, Langslet G, Hovingh GK, et al. Anacetrapib as lipid-modifying therapy in patients with heterozygous familial hypercholesterolaemia (REALIZE): a randomised, double-blind, placebo-controlled, phase 3 study. Lancet. 2015;385(9983):2153–61.

[145] Tavori H, Fan D, Blakemore JL, Yancey PG, Ding L, Linton MF, et al. Serum proprotein convertase subtilisin/kexin type 9 and cell surface low-density lipoprotein receptor: evidence for a reciprocal regulation. Circulation. 2013;127(24):2403–13.

[146] Pinkosky SL, Filippov S, Srivastava RA, Hanselman JC, Bradshaw CD, Hurley TR, et al. AMP-activated protein kinase and ATP-citrate lyase are two distinct molecular targets for ETC-1002, a novel small molecule regulator of lipid and carbohydrate metabolism. J Lipid Res. 2013;54(1):134–51.

[147] Ballantyne CM, Davidson MH, Macdougall DE, Bays HE, Dicarlo LA, Rosenberg NL, et al. Efficacy and safety of a novel dual modulator of adenosine triphosphate-citrate lyase and adenosine monophosphate-activated protein kinase in patients with hypercholesterolemia: results of a multicenter, randomized, double-blind, placebo-controlled, parallel-group trial. J Am Coll Cardiol. 2013;62(13):1154–62.

[148] Sirtori CR, Calabresi L, Franceschini G, Baldassarre D, Amato M, Johansson J, et al. Cardiovascular status of carriers of the Apolipoprotein A-I milano mutant. The Limone sul Garda Study. Circulation. 2001;103(15):1949–54.

[149] Nissen SE, Tsunoda T, Tuzcu EM, Schoenhagen P, Cooper CJ, Yasin M, et al. Effect of recombinant ApoA-I Milano on coronary atherosclerosis in patients with acute coronary syndromes: a randomized controlled trial. JAMA. 2003;290(17):2292–300.

[150] Karabina SA, Ninio E. Plasma PAF-acetylhydrolase: an unfulfilled promise? Biochim Biophys Acta. 2006;1761(11):1351–8.

[151] Collaboration L-PS. Thompson A, Gao P, Orfei L, Watson S, Di Angelantonio E, Kaptoge S, et al. Lipoprotein-associated phospholipase A2 and risk of coronary disease, stroke, and mortality: collaborative analysis of 32 prospective studies. Lancet. 2010;375(9725): 1536–44.

[152] Investigators S, White HD, Held C, Stewart R, Tarka E, Brown R, et al. Darapladib for preventing ischemic events in stable coronary heart disease. N Engl J Med. 2014;370(18): 1702–11.

Chapter 6

Cholesterol Lowering in Cancer Prevention and Therapy

Chunfa Huang and Carl E. Freter

Additional information is available at the end of the chapter

http://dx.doi.org/10.5772/65025

Abstract

The accumulation of cholesterol in cancer cells and tumor tissues promotes cell growth, proliferation, and migration as well as tumor progression. Cholesterol synthesis is catalyzed by a series of enzymatic reactions. Regulation of these key enzymes can control cholesterol synthesis and modulate cellular cholesterol levels in the cells. Meanwhile, controlling cholesterol transportation, absorption, and depletion could also significantly reduce cellular cholesterol levels. The current evidence supports that cholesterol lowering agents, beyond the expected cholesterol-lowering properties, also display an important anticancer activity in reducing cancer cell growth, proliferation and migration, and inducing apoptosis in a variety of cancer cells. Understanding the mechanisms of cholesterol metabolism and cholesterol lowering could potentially benefit cancer patients in cancer prevention and treatment.

Keywords: cholesterol metabolism, cholesterol-lowering agents, cancer, prevention, therapy

1. Introduction

Cholesterol is an essential component of cellular membrane. It serves as a spacer between the hydrocarbon chains, functions as dynamic glue during membrane assembly, and plays a crucial role in the stability, architecture, dynamics, and function of cellular membrane [1, 2]. In addition, cholesterol is involved in vesicle trafficking and transmembrane receptor signaling [3–6]. Meanwhile, cholesterol itself is also as a precursor of steroid hormones and sterols in the steroidogenesis [6–8]. The vesicle trafficking, receptor-mediated signaling, and steroidogenesis further lead to specific biological responses and regulate different cellular functions such as membrane biogenesis, cell growth, proliferation, apoptosis and migration, as well as tumor progression [6–8].

Due to the key physiological roles that cholesterol plays, the circulating and cellular cholesterol levels in our body are tightly regulated by a physiological balance of cholesterol biosynthesis, cholesterol catabolism, cholesterol transportation (influx and efflux), dietary cholesterol absorption, and cholesterol depletion. Higher cholesterol, also known as hypercholesterolemia, is a risk factor for a variety of human diseases such as cardiovascular diseases, dyslipidemia, Alzheimer's disease, HIV dyslipidemia, chronic inflammation, and developing diabetes. Earlier data also indicates that accelerated cholesterol metabolism and elevated cholesterol levels contribute to the hallmarks of cancer development and malignant transformation [9–15]. Cancer cells need excess cholesterol and intermediates of the cholesterol biosynthetic pathway to maintain a high level of cell growth and proliferation. Meanwhile, cholesterol is capable of regulating multiple signaling pathways involved in carcinogenesis, cancer cell migration, and tumor progression and is also involved in chemosensitivity and chemotherapy resistance of cancer cells [9–19]. It is very important to understand cholesterol as an important factor contributing to carcinogenesis and tumor progression and to elucidate the regulation of cholesterol metabolism as a new strategy for searching cancer prevention and therapy drugs.

2. Cell biology of cholesterol

2.1. De novo cholesterol biosynthesis

Cholesterol is a 27-carbon and tetracyclic ring steroid that is catalyzed by a series of more than 26 separate enzymatic reactions in several subcellular compartments [20, 21]. The de novo biosynthesis can be considered as five major steps: (1) From acetyl-CoA to 3-hydroxy-3-methylglutaryl coenzyme A (HMG-CoA): the acetyl-CoA can be derived from the oxidation of fatty acids or synthesized from cytosolic acetate precursors (metabolites or taken up from dietary or exogenous sources), and three acetyl-CoAs condense to form acetoacetyl-CoA by acetoacetyl-CoA acetyltransferases or thiolase and then HMG-CoA by HMG-CoA synthase. (2) The formation of mevalonate: HMG-CoA is reduced to mevalonate by HMG-CoA reductase, a rate-limiting and irreversible step in the metabolic pathway that produces cholesterol and other isoprenoids. (3) From mevalonate to isopentenyl pyrophosphate (IPP): mevalonate is further converted to IPP through two phosphorylation steps and one decarboxylation step. This conversion is involved in seven different enzymes (mevalonate-3-kinase, mevalonate-5-kinase, mevalonate-3-phosphate-5-kinase, phosphomevalonate kinase, mevalonate-5-phosphate decarboxylase, mevalonate pyrophosphate decarboxylase, and isopentenyl phosphate kinase) via different avenues. (4) From IPP to squalene: three molecules of IPP further condense to form a farnesyl pyrophosphate (FPP) and two molecules of FPP then condense to form squalene. The enzymes involved in the process are IPP isomerase, farnesyl-diphosphate synthase, and squalene synthase. (5) From squalene to lanosterol to cholesterol: the oxidation of squalene by squalene epoxidase forms 2,3-oxidosqualene which is further cyclized to lanosterol by squalene oxidocyclase. Lanosterol is finally converted to cholesterol by a series of demethylations, desaturations, isomerizations, and reductions. Demethylation reactions produce zymosterol as an intermediate and further converted to cholesterol by at least two pathways that differ in the order of the desaturations, isomerizations, and reductions (**Figure 1**) [22–27].

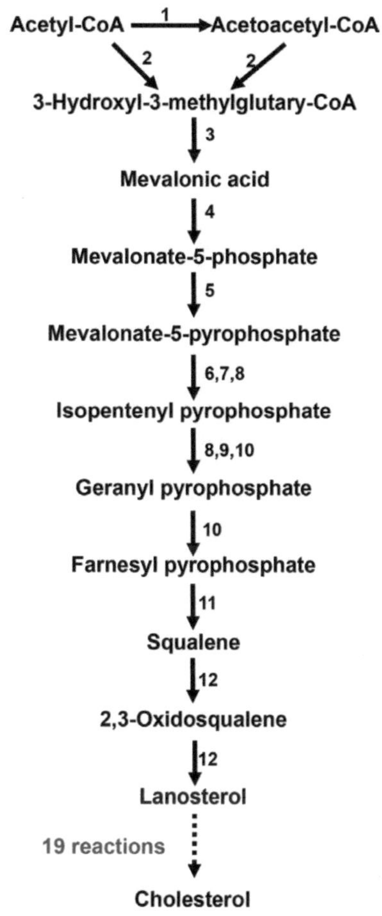

Figure 1. Scheme of the cholesterol biosynthesis pathway. (1) Thiolases or acetyl-coenzyme A acetyltransferases, (2) hydroxy-3-methylglutaryl-CoA synthase, (3) hydroxy-3-methylglutaryl-CoA reductase, (4) mevalonate-3-kinase or mevalonate-5-kinase, (5) mevalonate-3-phosphate-5-kinase or phosphomevalonate kinase, (6) mevalonate-5-phosphate decarboxylase, (7) mevalonate pyrophosphate decarboxylase, (8) isopentenyl phosphate kinase, (9) isopentenyl pyrophosphate isomerase, (10) farnesyl-diphosphate synthase, (11) squalene synthase, (12) squalene monooxygenase or squalene epoxidase, and 19 reactions are included multiple demethylations, desaturations, isomerizations, and reductions.

2.2. Cholesterol homeostasis

Cholesterol is a vital lipid and plays well-described biochemical roles and diverse functions at cellular level [1–3]. The homeostasis of cholesterol is among the most intensely regulated processes in our body. High cholesterol is a risk factor to numerous pathologies such as cardiovascular disease, atherosclerosis, dyslipidemia, and neurodegenerative diseases and is associated with the development of diabetes and cancer. Cholesterol homeostasis is achieved through intricate mechanisms involving biosynthesis, catabolism, dietary absorption, transportation (influx or efflux), and depletion (**Figure 2**) [28–32]. Slightly less than half of cholesterol in our body derives from de novo biosynthesis every day. The liver is the dominant site of cholesterol biosynthesis, and in vivo liver cholesterol production has been estimated at 1–2 g/day. Cholesterol is synthesized in liver and then secreted as circulating lipoproteins into bloodstream. The intestine and skin are also very important for cholesterol synthesis [33–35]. Although the majority of cholesterol sources comes from cholesterol biosynthesis, it is under feedback regulation. The absorption of cholesterol mainly derives from three sources: diet, bile, and intestinal epithelial sloughing. The average intake of cholesterol in the Western diet is approximately 300–500 mg per day. Bile is estimated to contribute nearly 800–1200 mg of cholesterol per day to the intraluminal pool. A third source of intraluminal cholesterol comes from the turnover of intestinal mucosal epithelium, which provides roughly 300 mg of cholesterol per day [36]. In cholesterol catabolism, the conversion of cholesterol into excretable bile acids represents the most relevant mechanism of irreversible elimination of cholesterol from the body, which plays a key role in hepatic and systemic cholesterol homeostasis. Under physiological conditions, approximately 300–400 mg of cholesterol is disposed in the liver daily [37]. Because peripheral cells do not catabolize the cholesterol molecule, there are two distinct mechanisms for maintaining cellular cholesterol homeostasis. One is the nonspecific classical pathway mediated by physicochemical diffusion of cholesterol through the aqueous phase and the other is cholesterol esterification on high-density lipoprotein (HDL) by lecithin: cholesterol acyltransferase reaction [38, 39]. The reaction is initiated by the interaction of lipid-free or lipid-poor apolipoproteins with cellular surface resulting in the assembly of HDL particles with phospholipid and cholesterol as well as extracellular cholesterol esterification mainly on HDL [40]. Furthermore, changing dietary style to control cholesterol absorption and using pharmaceutical drugs to inhibit several key enzymes in cholesterol synthesis can also significantly reduce the level of cellular cholesterol. All of these pharmaceutical drugs and dietary style have been commonly used for keeping a healthy life and preventing heart disease [41–44].

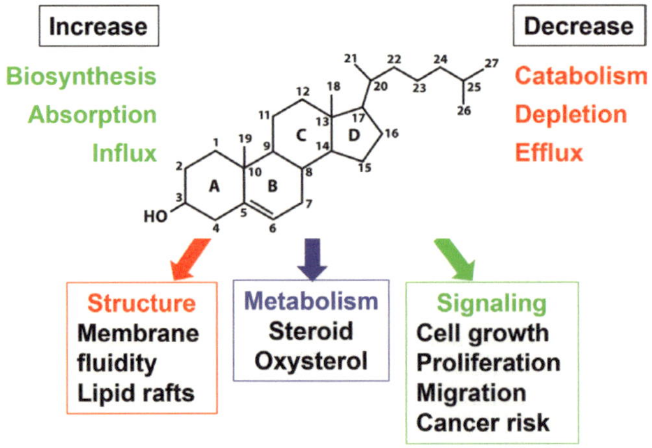

Figure 2. Cholesterol homeostasis and functions. Cholesterol homeostasis is tightly regulated in our body and can be achieved through intricate mechanisms involved in biosynthesis, dietary absorption, transportation (influx or efflux), catabolism, and depletion. The functions of cholesterol are composed of distinct membrane, control membrane fluidity and protein recruitment, produce steroid and oxysterol, and are involved in cell signaling to regulate cell growth, proliferation, and migration.

2.3. Biological functions of cholesterol

Disruption to cholesterol homeostasis leads to a variety of diseases such as coronary heart disease, atherosclerosis, and metabolic syndrome as well as cancer [9–19, 45–51]. This indicates that cholesterol plays a crucial role in the regulation of cellular function (**Figure 2**). In the cells, cholesterol is mandatory for cellular growth and serves as one of the necessary building blocks for new membranes demanded by dividing cells during proliferation. Cell membranes have been recognized as heterogeneous structures composed of distinct membrane microdomains with different proteins and lipids. Lipid rafts, cholesterol-rich domains, play an important platform as a signaling station for many cellular processes, including membrane sorting and trafficking, cell polarization, and signal transduction [52–56]. Cholesterol promotes cell proliferation by inducing the activation of the AKT and/or the ERK signaling pathway as well as Ca^{2+} channel [57–60] and cell migration by increasing the activity of calpain that is also Ca^{2+} dependent [61, 62] and is also involved in Hedgehog processing, diffusion, and reception [63, 64]. Cholesterol can be converted to steroid hormones which activate nuclear receptors and thus help to control metabolism, inflammation, immune functions, salt and water balance, the development of sexual characteristics, and the ability to withstand illness and injury [65, 66]. Meanwhile, the metabolites of cholesterol such as hydroxycholesterols play multiple biological functions in the body [67, 68]. Cholesterol also contributes to chemotherapy resistance which leads to treat failure [11–14]. Taken together, cholesterol is tightly associated with cancer cell growth, proliferation and therapy.

3. The balance of cholesterol and cancer

Cholesterol accumulation in cancer cells and tumor tissues was discovered in cancer cells and tumor tissues started in earlier 1900s [12, 69, 70]. Since then, researchers have studied the relationship between cellular cholesterol and cancer in depth. Recent epidemiological studies suggest the correlation between serum cholesterol level and the risk of certain types of cancer [15, 71–74]. It is difficult to draw conclusions from epidemiological studies on whether cholesterol is a key factor of cancer incidence because of of their intrinsic limitations. On the other hand, experimental evidence from cell and animal models indicates that cholesterol plays a promotional role in cancer cell growth and cancer development and progression [57–60]. These findings support the notion that lowering cholesterol level may be a useful and effective strategy for cancer prevention and a therapeutic potential for cancer treatment.

3.1. Lowering cholesterol level

As described above, cholesterol homeostasis is controlled by its biosynthesis, catabolism, dietary absorption, transportation, and depletion [28–32]. Among these, cholesterol biosynthesis and absorption with low-density lipoprotein (LDL) receptor (LDLR) which mediates the endocytosis of cholesterol-rich LDL are key to elevate cellular cholesterol. By contrast, there are also two common avenues to achieve cholesterol lowering: (1) pharmacological treatment which inhibits cholesterol biosynthesis [41–45] and (2) dietary control that reduces cholesterol absorption [36, 75]. Meanwhile, cholesterol metabolite, 27-hydroxycholesterol, and other oxysterols can activate the liver X receptors (LXR), resulting in a reduction of intracellular cholesterol [76–78]. Modulation of LXR and their downstream targets has appeared to be involved in cholesterol and lipid metabolism in response to changes in cellular cholesterol status [76–78]. This also draws attention to the therapeutic interest of developing LXR agonists as a bona fide therapeutic approach in cancer treatment. The cross talk of LDLR-SREBP (sterol regulatory element-binding protein) signaling and LXR signaling in the regulation of cholesterol metabolism is potential as a new strategy to develop cancer therapeutic drugs and treatment regimen.

3.2. Cholesterol-lowering drugs

There are many different agents that can inhibit cholesterol biosynthesis at different enzymatic steps or reduce cholesterol level by different regulation pathways. **Table 1** summaries the targets and effects of different cholesterol-lowering agents. Statins, first marketed in 1987, are the most common drugs to lower cholesterol level. As structural analogues of HMG-CoA, statins inhibit HMG-CoA reductase to block the conversion of HMG-CoA to mevalonic acid in a rate-limiting step of cholesterol biosynthesis. Up to date, a number of different compounds in this class drugs have been developed: atorvastatin (Lipitor), cerivastatin (Baycol; withdrawn from the market in 2001), fluvastatin (Lescol), lovastatin (Mevacor), mevastatin (Compactin), pitavastatin (Livalo), pravastatin (Pravachol or Selektine), rosuvastatin (Crestor), and simvastatin (Zocor). They are effective for treating cardiovascular disease, atherosclerosis, dyslipoproteinemia, and liver disease [79–81] and are also recommended for those who do not meet their lipid-lowering goals through diet and lifestyle changes. Statins are also considered as an anticancer agent to prevent and treat cancer patients [42–44]. Because of multiple side effects of statins, such as muscle pain, increased risk of diabetes mellitus, and abnormalities in liver enzyme tests, many other enzymes that are involved in cholesterol biosynthetic pathway beyond HMG-CoA reductase are also being considered as targets for developing cholesterol-lowering drugs. These drugs include bisphosphonates which inhibit farnesyl-diphosphate synthase [82] and lonafarnib (SCH66366) and tipifarnib (R115777) which inhibit farnesyltransferase [83]. YM-53601, RPR-107393, and TAK-475 (Lapaquistat) can inhibit squalene synthase [84–86], and Ro 48-8071, BIBB515, and terbinafine (Lamisil) are potent inhibitors of 2,3-oxidosqualene cyclase or squalene epoxidase [87–89]. These agents are used in clinic and in clinic trials.

In addition, several another classes of compounds which can lower cholesterol level via different molecular mechanisms have recently been developed. Ezetimibe (Zetia), a cholesterol uptake-blocking drug, prevents cholesterol absorption from dietary intake [90]. Fibrate drugs (Gemfibrozil, Tricor, Atromid-S), an activator of peroxisome proliferator-activated receptor α (PPARα), can reduce very-low-density lipoprotein (VLDL) - and LDL-containing apoprotein B and increase HDL-containing apoprotein AI and AII [91, 92]. Cholestyramine, colestipol, and colesevelam, bile acid sequestrants, can remove bile acids from the body and further convert more plasma cholesterol to bile acids to reduce cholesterol level [93, 94]. Some other cholesterol-lowering agents are also on the market or available for research. Acyl-CoA:cholesteryl acyltransferase inhibitor (avasimibe or CI-1011) induces cholesterol 7-α-hydroxylase and increases bile acid synthesis [95]. Green tea or catechins can inhibit the intestinal absorption of dietary lipids [96]. Lomitapide (Juxtapid) inhibits the microsomal triglyceride transfer protein required for VLDL assembly and secretion [97]. Mipomersen is a second-generation antisense oligonucleotide targeted to human apolipoprotein B-100 which is the structural core of LDL cholesterol [98]. Anacetrapib is a novel inhibitor of cholesteryl ester transfer protein [99]. Evolocumab (AMG145) and alirocumab are monoclonal antibodies which inactivate the proprotein convertase subtilisin/kexin type 9 (PCSK9) and lower LDL level [100, 101]. Dynasore reduces labile cholesterol in the plasma membrane [102]. Some of these cholesterol-lowering drugs have demonstrated their anticancer property and have the potential of cancer pharmacological prevention [41–45].

Agents	Targets	Effects	References
Statins	HMG-CoA reductase	Block the conversion of HMG-CoA to mevalonic acid	[79–81]
Bisphosphonate	FPP synthase	Attenuate the formation of FPP	[82]
SCH66366 R115777	Farnesyltransferase	Reduce adding a farnesyl group to proteins	[83]
YM-53601 RPR-107393 TAK-475	Squalene synthase	Inhibit the conversion of FPP to squalene	[84–86]
Ro 48-8071	2,3-Oxidosqualene synthase	Block the formation of 2,3 oxidosqualene	[87, 88]
BIBB515 Terbinafine	Squalene epoxidase		
Ezetimibe Catechins	Cholesterol absorption	Block cholesterol uptake in the small intestine	[89, 90]
Gemfibrozil Tricor Atromid-S	PPARα	Reduce VLDL and LDL level	[91, 92]
Cholestyramine Colesevelam and the conversion of cholesterol to bile acid Colestipol	Bile acid sequestrants	Increase bile acid removal	[93, 94]
Avasimibe CI-1011	ACAT	Increase cholesterol oxidation and bile acid synthesis	[95, 96]
Lomitapide	Triglyceride transfer protein	Reduce VLDL assembly and secretion	[97]
Mipomersen	Apolipoprotein B-100	Reduce LDL level	[98]
Evolocumab Alirocumab	PCSK9 antibody	Inactivate PCSK9 and lower LDL level	[99, 100]
Dynasore	Dynamin	Reduce membrane cholesterol	[101]

*PPARα, peroxisome proliferator-activated receptor α; ACAT, Acyl-CoA:cholesteryl acyltransferase.

Table 1. Targets and effects of different cholesterol-lowering agents.

3.3. Anticancer property of cholesterol-lowering drugs

Accumulating evidence supports that deregulation of any steps in cell growth, proliferation, and migration may result in cell malignant transformation. More than a century ago, cholesterol was observed to accumulate in malignant tissues [69]. Now, more and more evidence shows that cholesterol plays a critical role in the regulation of cancer cell growth and proliferation and tumor progression [8, 10–18, 70]. The key regulators in cholesterol metabolism attract many researchers around the world to search for novel anticancer agents. Based on cholesterol biofunctions and experimental data, the role of cholesterol-lowering drugs may not limit on the property of LDL-cholesterol lowering but may also be involved in the prevention or treatment of cancer. Statins are the most common cholesterol-lowering drugs and are also the most studied drugs. Whether statins exhibit anticancer properties is based on experimental studies, epidemiological studies, and clinical studies. In experimental studies, statins reduce a variety of cancer cell viability (**Figure 3**) [75, 103–105]. The epidemiologic data also support that statins reduce the incidence of gastric cancer, breast cancer, advanced prostate cancer, colorectal cancer, and cholangiocarcinoma [105–109]. However, there are also some studies that do not support the association of statin use with cancer risk [110, 111]. In clinical studies, statins can significantly reduce prostate cancer-specific mortality and reduce the risk of biochemical recurrence among the patients treated with radiation therapy [112] and are also associated with improved survival in patients with metastatic renal cell carcinoma [113]. So far, statins show some promising results in certain types of cancer. The potential of statins in modern cancer prevention and treatment is very promising. Meanwhile, it is also important to search other cholesterol-lowering agents that are more effective and reduce adverse side effects. Some of these agents have already been studied at the different stages [89, 114].

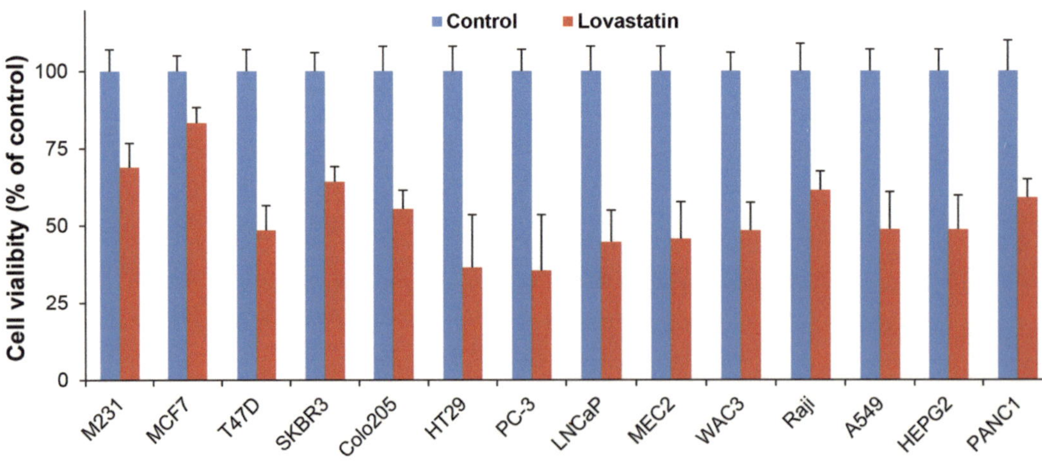

Figure 3. Treatment of lovastatin reduces cell viability in different cancer cell lines. Different cancer cells were cultured in 96-well plates and treated with 10 μM lovastatin for 3 days; the samples analyzed cell viability by MTT assay (n = 16). The values of lovastatin treatment were statistically different from the controls. $P < 0.05$. M231, MDA-MB-231.

3.4. Molecular mechanism of anticancer properties of cholesterol-lowering drugs

Expression of HMG-CoA reductase gene can be regulated by genetic or dietary interaction [115], in which it is transcriptionally regulated by endoplasmic reticulum-based transcription factor, SREBP-2 [116], or high-fat diet feeding [117]. Statins inhibit HMG-CoA reductase to block cholesterol biosynthesis which attenuate cell proliferation and arrest cell cycle progression by interrupting growth-promoting signals and involving in RAS/RAF/MEK/ERK, PI3K/AKT/mTOR and Wnt/β-catenin signaling cascades [118, 119]. Statins also selectively induce proapoptotic potential in tumor cells and synergistically enhance proapoptotic potential of several cytotoxic agents. The mechanism for this effect has been demonstrated by disrupted binding of RhoA inhibitor GDIα which leads to increased levels of GTP-bound forms of RhoA, Rac1, and cdc42 proteins.These proteins induce apoptosis 1) by suppression of anti-apoptotic proteins such as Bcl2 or activation of the superoxide-activated JNK pathway [120] or 2) by inhibiting Akt/mTOR pathway and inducing programmed cell death 4 expression in renal cell cancer cells [121]. Statins alter the angiogenic potential of cells by modulating apoptosis inhibitory effects of VEGF and decrease secretion of metalloproteases and suppress the rate of activation of multiple coagulation factors and thus prevent coagulation-mediated angiogenesis [122]. Statins suppress the Rho/Rho-associated coiled-coil-containing protein kinase pathways, thereby inhibiting cell migration, invasion, adhesion, and metastasis [123]. Other cholesterol-lowering agents have not been widely studied as statins. However, all cholesterol-lowering agents could affect membrane composition, in particular cholesterol-rich domain, termed lipid rafts. Membrane lipid rafts are highly ordered membrane domains that are enriched in cholesterol, sphingolipids, and gangliosides and selectively recruit certain classes of proteins (a large number of cancer-related signaling and adhesion molecules) and act as major modulators of membrane geometry, lateral movement of molecules, and traffic and signal transduction [52, 54]. Cholesterol-lowering drugs lead to membrane cholesterol depletion which could disrupt membrane lipid rafts, block the adhesion and migration processes of cancer cells, and induce cancer cell apoptosis [124, 125].

4. Cholesterol-lowering drugs in cancer prevention and therapy

A growing body of evidence from cell biology and animal models has strongly demonstrated the anticancer activity of cholesterol-lowering drugs such as statins [7, 83–89, 104–108]. Epidemiological studies also suggest an anticancer effect of statins evidenced by the reductions of cancer incidence and cancer-related mortality, although the association between statin use and cancer incidence based on different cancer remains controversial from different laboratories around the world. Statins as part of pharmacological cancer prevention and chemotherapy have generated interest in the oncology community and have been investigated in a variety of cancers at early and late stages and in the combination with chemotherapy and radiation therapy. Here, we summarize the current data that statin use affects cancer incidence and therapy.

Study	No. of subjects/ studies	Results	References
Bonovas, 2008	12 studies	No significant relationship between statins and pancreatic cancer risk	[129]
Khurana, 2007	483,733	Protective against the development of pancreatic cancer	[130]
Lin, 2016	19,727	Prevent *H. pylori*-associated gastric cancer	[105]
Singh, 2013	11 studies	Prevent gastric cancer risk in both Asian and Western population	[131]
Tsan, 2012	33,413	Reduce the risk for hepatocellular carcinoma in HBV-infected patients	[132]
Chen, 2015	2,053	Decrease hepatocellular carcinoma in diabetic patients	[133]
Zhang, 2013	13 studies	No association between statin use and risk of bladder cancer	[134]
Peng, 2015	3,174	Reduce the risk of cholangiocarcinoma	[108]
Yi, 2014	20 studies	Preventive effects against hematological malignancies	[135]
Pradelli, 2015	14 studies	Negatively associated with all hematological malignancies	[136]
Wang, 2013	20 studies	Nonsignificant association between statin users and lung cancer risk	[137]
Bansal, 2012	27 studies	Reduce the risk of total and advanced prostate cancer	[138]
Jacobs, 2007	55,454	Reduce the risk of advanced prostate cancer	[109]
Undela, 2012	24 studies	Do not support that statins have a protective effect against breast cancer	[139]
Lytras, 2014	40 studies	Do not support that statin users reduce the risk of colorectal cancer	[140]
Setoguchi, 2007	24,439	No effect in the risk of colorectal, lung, or breast cancer in older patients	[141]
Kuoppala, 2008	42 studies	No effect on the incidence of lung, breast, or prostate cancer Protect from stomach and liver cancer and from lymphoma Increase the incidence of both melanoma and nonmelanoma skin cancer	[142]

Table 2. Effect of statins on cancer incidence.

4.1. Cholesterol-lowering drugs in cancer prevention

Cholesterol is accumulated in different solid tumors and cancer cells [12, 69–71, 126, 127], raising questions concerning the role of cholesterol in cancer cell growth, proliferation, and migration as well as tumor progression [57–61]. Although cholesterol-lowering drugs have also been shown to possess an important antitumor activity that reduces cell growth, proliferation, and migration through ERK-mediated and Akt-mediated signaling pathways and is capable of inducing apoptosis through extrinsic and intrinsic pathways using different cancer cells as models [43–45, 75, 78, 104, 118–123], it is still unclear whether statins are suitable to prevent the incidence of cancer. More than a hundred of epidemiological studies around the world have been performed to evaluate the effect of statin on the risk of cancer incidence [105, 108, 109, 126–142]. These studies have been focused on statin type, potency, lipophilic or hydrophobicity status, and duration of use. Due to the limitation of epidemiological studies with the patients different in age, sex, living regions, and life style, the results are controversial. **Table 2** summarizes the association of cancer risk and statin use in pancreatic cancer, gastric cancer, liver cancer, lung cancer, bladder cancer, breast cancer, prostate cancer, colorectal cancer, blood cancer, and other malignancies. The clinical studies have provided conflicting data regarding whether statins may reduce or may be no effect on the risk of cancer. It is clear that current data cannot rule out the association of statin use with the risk of some cancers. Analyses of larger numbers of cases, subgroup design (participant ethnicity or confounder adjustment), randomized controlled trials, and high-quality cohort studies with longer duration of follow-up are needed to further confirm this association. Meanwhile, we also need to study cancer patient genetic mutations and determine whether the effect of statins on cancer prevention and therapy is associated with genetic mutation. It is clear that defining the underlying mechanisms of how cholesterol lowering contributes to cancer prevention and the search for other cholesterol-lowering agents with better outcome has emerged as future objectives. Whether cholesterol-lowering agents are used in cancer prevention will be based on the analysis of responses to these agents with cancer patient genetic information.

4.2. Cholesterol-lowering drugs in cancer treatment

Cholesterol is implicated in various cellular processes including the involvement of cell proliferation/apoptosis balance regulation in various types of cancers. Statins and other cholesterol-lowering agents are very common and effective medication used in preventing heart disease in those with high cholesterol, but no history of heart disease. The anticancer activity of these drugs has also attracted oncologists to consider whether cholesterol-lowering drugs can be a tool for cancer treatment. A variety of studies have focused on the effect of statins alone or in combination with other chemo- or/and immune-therapeutic drugs or radiation therapy on the treatment of different cancer patients. McKay et al. [113] showed some promising data that statin use improved survival in patients with metastatic renal cell carcinoma. Raval et al. found that statin significantly reduced the prostate cancer-specific mortality and improved the biochemical recurrence in certain subgroup of men with prostate cancer [112]. Song et al. found that statin use also reduces biochemical recurrence in men with prostate cancer after radical prostatectomy [143]. Statin use is related to reductions in overall and cancer-specific mortality [144] and associated with longer rates of survival [145] in colorectal cancer survivors. Two recent studies indicate that statin use is associated with improved overall survival in patients with resectable pancreatic ductal adenocarcinoma [146, 147]. Statin use also improves overall survival among patients undergoing resection for pancreatic cancer [148]. Lipophilic statins are associated with a reduced risk of breast cancer recurrence and inflammatory breast cancer [149]. Because statins negatively interfere with CD-20 and rituximab-mediated activity, statins have a negatively effect on clinical outcome in patients with rituximab-treated leukemia [150]. No association of statin use with patient survivals was also reported from colorectal cancer study [151]. Future studies are needed to further evaluate which cancer patients may benefit from statin treatment, what the best treatment is, and which cholesterol-lowering drugs are better to use in cancer treatment.

5. Concluding remarks and future perspectives

Cholesterol is tightly regulated by a physiological balance of cholesterol metabolism (biosynthesis and degradation), dietary absorption, transportation (efflux and influx), and depletion.

Importantly, cholesterol is accumulated in cancer cells and tumor tissues and is implicated in various cellular processes including cell growth, proliferation, and migration. The increase and decrease in cellular and circulating cholesterol levels have demonstrated the involvement of cell proliferation/apoptosis balance regulation. This chapter reviewed our current understanding of how cholesterol metabolism contributes to cancer development and progression and cholesterol-lowering drugs may be associated with the therapeutic potential of cancer prevention and treatment. Current evidence cannot exclude the relevance of cancer risk with statin use as seen in a variety of studies. Whether the genetic mutations of cancer patients are associated with the response of statins is also unknown. It is clear that more studies are needed to better characterize potential statin-mediated mechanisms that prevent cancer incidence. On the other hand, statins alone or used in combination with certain anticancer drugs or radiation therapy can improve survival in patients with several different tumors. Further research using large cohort studies in different cancers is needed to clarify these issues. In addition, searching for novel classes of cholesterol-lowering drugs with more effects and less side effects could provide new therapeutic options for cancer prevention and therapy.

Acknowledgements

Conflict of interest: The authors declare no conflict of interest.

Author details

Chunfa Huang* and Carl E. Freter

*Address all correspondence to: chunfahuang@slu.edu

Division of Hematology and Oncology, Department of Internal Medicine, and Cancer Center, Saint Louis University, Saint Louis, Missouri, United States of America

References

[1] Grouleff J, Irudayam SJ, Skeby KK, Schiøtt B. The influence of cholesterol on membrane protein structure, function, and dynamics studied by molecular dynamics simulations. Biochim Biophys Acta. 2015; 1848:1783-95.

[2] Mesmin B, Maxfield FR. Intracellular sterol dynamics. Biochim Biophys Acta. 2009; 1791:636-45.

[3] Wüstner D, Solanko K. How cholesterol interacts with proteins and lipids during its intracellular transport. Biochim Biophys Acta. 2015; 1848:1908-26.

[4] Sengupta D, Chattopadhyay A. Molecular dynamics simulations of GPCR-cholesterol interaction: an emerging paradigm. Biochim Biophys Acta. 2015; 1848:1775-82.

[5] Du X, Brown AJ, Yang H. Novel mechanisms of intracellular cholesterol transport: oxysterol-binding proteins and membrane contact sites. Curr Opin Cell Biol. 2015; 35:37-42.

[6] Papadopoulos V, Aghazadeh Y, Fan J, Campioli E, Zirkin B, Midzak A. Translocator protein-mediated pharmacology of cholesterol transport and steroidogenesis. Mol Cell Endocrinol. 2015; 408:90-8.

[7] Issop L, Rone MB, Papadopoulos V. Organelle plasticity and interactions in cholesterol transport and steroid biosynthesis. Mol Cell Endocrinol. 2013; 371:34-46.

[8] Simons K, Ikonen E. How cells handle cholesterol. Science. 2000; 290:1721-6.

[9] Cruz PM, Mo H, McConathy WJ, Sabnis N, Lacko AG. The role of cholesterol metabolism and cholesterol transport in carcinogenesis: a review of scientific findings, relevant to future cancer therapeutics. Front Pharmacol. 2013; 4:119.

[10] Nelson ER, Chang CY, McDonnell DP. Cholesterol and breast cancer pathophysiology. Trends Endocrinol Metab. 2014; 25:649-55.

[11] Danilo C, Frank PG. Cholesterol and breast cancer development. Curr Opin Pharmacol. 2012; 12:677-82.

[12] Krycer JR, Brown AJ. Cholesterol accumulation in prostate cancer: a classic observation from a modern perspective. Biochim Biophys Acta. 2013; 1835:219-29.

[13] Drabkin HA, Gemmill RM. Cholesterol and the development of clear-cell renal carcinoma. Curr Opin Pharmacol. 2012; 12:742-50.

[14] Jacobs RJ, Voorneveld PW, Kodach LL, Hardwick JC. Cholesterol metabolism and colorectal cancers. Curr Opin Pharmacol. 2012; 12:690-5.

[15] Murai T. Cholesterol lowering: role in cancer prevention and treatment. Biol Chem. 2015; 396:1-11.

[16] Silvente-Poirot S, Poirot M. Cancer. Cholesterol and cancer, in the balance. Science. 2014; 343:1445-6.

[17] Pelton K, Freeman MR, Solomon KR: Cholesterol and prostate cancer. Curr Opin Pharmacol 2012; 12:751-759.

[18] Gorin A, Gabitova L, Astsaturov I: Regulation of cholesterol biosynthesis and cancer signaling. Curr Opin Pharmacol. 2012; 12:710-716.

[19] Hilvo M, Denkert C, Lehtinen L, Muller B, Brockmoller S, Seppanen-Laakso T, Budczies J, Bucher E, Yetukuri L, Castillo S, Berg E, Nygren H, Sysi-Aho M, Griffin JL, Fiehn O,

Loibl S, Richter-Ehrenstein C, Radke C, Hyötyläinen T, Kallioniemi O, Iljin K, Oresic M: Novel theranostic opportunities offered by characterization of altered membrane lipid metabolism in breast cancer progression. Cancer Res 2011; 71:3236-3245.

[20] Nelson DL and Cox MM eds. Lehninger Principles of Biochemistry. 6th edition, 2012, W.H. Freeman & Company, New York.

[21] Berg JM, Tymockzo JL and Stryer L. Biochemistry. 7th edition, 2012, W.H. Freeman & Company, New York.

[22] Porter FD, Herman GE. Malformation syndromes caused by disorders of cholesterol synthesis. J Lipid Res. 2011; 52:6-34.

[23] Fu Z, Voynova NE, Herdendorf TJ, Miziorko HM, Kim JJ. Biochemical and structural basis for feedback inhibition of mevalonate kinase and isoprenoid metabolism. Biochemistry 2008; 47: 3715-24.

[24] Gaylor JL. Membrane-bound enzymes of cholesterol synthesis from lanosterol. Biochem Biophys Res Commun 2002; 292:1139-46.

[25] Goldstein JL, Brown MS. Regulation of the mevalonate pathway. Nature 1990; 343:425-30.

[26] Miziorko HM. Enzymes of the mevalonate pathway of isoprenoid biosynthesis. Arch Biochem Biophys 2011; 505:131-43.

[27] Houten SM, Frenkel J, Waterham HR. Isoprenoid biosynthesis in hereditary periodic fever syndromes and inflammation. Cell Mol Life Sci 2003; 60:1118-34.

[28] Luu W, Sharpe LJ, Gelissen IC, Brown AJ. The role of signalling in cellular cholesterol homeostasis. IUBMB Life. 2013; 65:675-84.

[29] van der Wulp MY, Verkade HJ, Groen AK. Regulation of cholesterol homeostasis. Mol Cell Endocrinol. 2013; 368:1-16.

[30] Goedeke L, Fernández-Hernando C. Regulation of cholesterol homeostasis. Cell Mol Life Sci. 2012; 69:915-30.

[31] Sharpe LJ, Cook EC, Zelcer N, Brown AJ. The UPS and downs of cholesterol homeostasis. Trends Biochem Sci. 2014; 39:527-35.

[32] Malgrange B, Varela-Nieto I, de Medina P, Paillasse MR. Targeting cholesterol homeostasis to fight hearing loss: a new perspective. Front Aging Neurosci. 2015; 7:3.

[33] Nestel PJ, Whyte HM, Goodman DS. Distribution and turnover of cholesterol in humans. J Clin Invest. 1969; 48:982-991.

[34] Nestel PJ. Cholesterol turnover in man. Adv Lipid Res. 1970; 8:1-39.

[35] Ho KJ, Taylor CB. Control mechanisms of cholesterol biosynthesis. Arch Pathol. 1970; 90:83-92.

[36] Wang DQ. Regulation of intestinal cholesterol absorption. Annu Rev Physiol. 2007; 69:221-48.

[37] Bertolotti M, Gabbi C, Anzivino C, Carulli L, Loria P, Carulli N. Nuclear receptors as potential molecular targets in cholesterol accumulation conditions: insights from evidence on hepatic cholesterol degradation and gallstone disease in humans. Curr Med Chem 2008; 15:2271–2284.

[38] Czarnecka H, Yokoyama S. Lecithin:cholesterol acyltransferase reaction on cellular lipid released by free apolipoprotein-mediated efflux. Biochemistry 1995; 34:4385-4392.

[39] Tomimoto S, Tsujita M, Okazaki M, Usui S, Tada T, Fukutomi T, Ito S, Itoh M, Yokoyama S. Effect of probucol in lecithin:cholesterol acyltransferase-deficient mice: inhibition of 2 independent cellular cholesterol-releasing pathways in vivo. Arterioscler Thromb Vasc Biol 2001; 21:394-400.

[40] Yokoyama S. Release of cellular cholesterol: molecular mechanism for cholesterol homeostasis in cells and in the body. Biochim Biophys Acta. 2000; 1529:231-44.

[41] Gumbs PD, Verschuren MW, Mantel-Teeuwisse AK, de Wit AG, de Boer A, Klungel OH. Economic evaluations of cholesterol-lowering drugs: a critical and systematic review. Pharmacoeconomics. 2007; 25:187-99.

[42] Alla VM, Agrawal V, DeNazareth A, Mohiuddin S, Ravilla S, Rendell M. A reappraisal of the risks and benefits of treating to target with cholesterol lowering drugs. Drugs. 2013; 73:1025-54

[43] Bardou M, Barkun A, Martel M. Effect of statin therapy on colorectal cancer. Gut. 2010; 59:1572-85.

[44] Sassano A, Platanias LC. Statins in tumor suppression. Cancer Lett. 2008; 260:11-9.

[45] Goldstein JL, Brown MS. A century of cholesterol and coronaries: from plaques to genes to statins. Cell. 2015; 161:161-72.

[46] Seo HS, Choi MH. Cholesterol homeostasis in cardiovascular disease and recent advances in measuring cholesterol signatures. J Steroid Biochem Mol Biol. 2015; 153:72-9.

[47] Varbo A, Nordestgaard BG. Remnant cholesterol and ischemic heart disease. Curr Opin Lipidol. 2014; 25:266-73.

[48] Tall AR, Yvan-Charvet L. Cholesterol, inflammation and innate immunity. Nat Rev Immunol. 2015; 15:104-16.

[49] Zhang J, Liu Q. Cholesterol metabolism and homeostasis in the brain. Protein Cell. 2015; 6:254-64.

[50] Leoni V, Caccia C. The impairment of cholesterol metabolism in Huntington disease. Biochim Biophys Acta. 2015; 1851:1095-105.

[51] Hannaoui S, Shim SY, Cheng YC, Corda E, Gilch S. Cholesterol balance in prion diseases and Alzheimer's disease. Viruses. 2014; 6:4505-35.

[52] Simons K, Toomre D. Lipid rafts and signal transduction. Nat Rev Mol Cell Biol. 2000; 1:31–39.

[53] Brown DA, London E. Functions of lipid rafts in biological membranes. Annu Rev Cell Dev Biol. 1998; 14:111–136.

[54] Mollinedo F, Gajate C. Lipid rafts as major platforms for signaling regulation in cancer. Adv Biol Regul. 2015; 57:130-46.

[55] Reeves VL, Thomas CM, Smart EJ. Lipid rafts, caveolae and GPI-linked proteins. Adv Exp Med Biol. 2012; 729:3-13.

[56] Lajoie P, Nabi IR. Lipid rafts, caveolae, and their endocytosis. Int Rev Cell Mol Biol. 2010; 282:135-63.

[57] Sun Y, Sukumaran P, Varma A, Derry S, Sahmoun AE, Singh BB. Cholesterol-induced activation of TRPM7 regulates cell proliferation, migration, and viability of human prostate cells. Biochim Biophys Acta. 2014; 1843:1839-50.

[58] dos Santos CR, Domingues G, Matias I, Matos J, Fonseca I, de Almeida JM, Dias S. LDL-cholesterol signaling induces breast cancer proliferation and invasion. Lipids Health Dis. 2014; 13:16.

[59] Xu F, Rychnovsky SD, Belani JD, Hobbs HH, Cohen JC, Rawson RB. Dual roles for cholesterol in mammalian cells. Proc Natl Acad Sci U S A. 2005; 102:14551-6.

[60] Chen BY, Wei JG, Wang YC, Yu J, Qian JX, Chen YM, Xu J. Effects of cholesterol on proliferation and functional protein expression in rabbit bile duct fibroblasts. World J Gastroenterol. 2004; 10:889-93.

[61] Franco SJ, Huttenlocher A. Regulating cell migration: calpains make the cut. J Cell Sci 2005; 118:3829-3838.

[62] Sukumaran P, Lof C, Pulli I, Kemppainen K, Viitanen T, Tornquist K. Significance of the transient receptor potential canonical 2 (TRPC2) channel in the regulation of rat thyroid FRTL-5 cell proliferation, migration, adhesion and invasion. Mol Cell Endocrinol 2013; 374:10–21.

[63] Riobo NA. Cholesterol and its derivatives in Sonic Hedgehog signaling and cancer. Curr Opin Pharmacol. 2012; 12:736-41.

[64] Callahan BP, Wang C. Hedgehog cholesterolysis: specialized gatekeeper to oncogenic signaling. Cancers (Basel). 2015; 7:2037-53.

[65] Sewer MB, Li D. Regulation of steroid hormone biosynthesis by the cytoskeleton. Lipids. 2008; 43:1109-15.

[66] Mani SK, Mermelstein PG, Tetel MJ, Anesetti G. Convergence of multiple mechanisms of steroid hormone action. Horm Metab Res. 2012; 44:569-76.

[67] Javitt NB. Biologic role(s) of the 25(R),26-hydroxycholesterol metabolic pathway. Biochim Biophys Acta. 2000; 1529:136-41.

[68] Ren S, Ning Y. Sulfation of 25-hydroxycholesterol regulates lipid metabolism, inflammatory responses, and cell proliferation. Am J Physiol Endocrinol Metab. 2014; 306:E123-30.

[69] White, C.P. On the occurrence of crystals in tumours. J Pathol Bacteriol. 1909; 13: 3-10.

[70] Clayman RV, Gonzalez R, Elliott AY, Gleason DE, Dempsey ME. Cholesterol accumulation in heterotransplanted renal cell cancer. J Urol. 1983; 129:621-4.

[71] Wang J, Wang WJ, Zhai L, Zhang DF. Association of cholesterol with risk of pancreatic cancer: a meta-analysis. World J Gastroenterol. 2015; 21:3711-9.

[72] Touvier M, Fassier P, His M, Norat T, Chan DS, Blacher J, Hercberg S, Galan P, Druesne-Pecollo N, Latino-Martel P. Cholesterol and breast cancer risk: a systematic review and meta-analysis of prospective studies. Br J Nutr. 2015; 114:347-57.

[73] Vílchez JA, Martínez-Ruiz A, Sancho-Rodríguez N, Martínez-Hernández P, Noguera-Velasco JA. The real role of prediagnostic high-density lipoprotein cholesterol and the cancer risk: a concise review. Eur J Clin Invest. 2014; 44:103-14.

[74] Freeman MR, Solomon KR. Cholesterol and prostate cancer. J Cell Biochem. 2004; 91:54-69.

[75] Kato S, Smalley S, Sadarangani A, Chen-Lin K, Oliva B, Brañes J, Carvajal J, Gejman R, Owen GI, Cuello M. Lipophilic but not hydrophilic statins selectively induce cell death in gynaecological cancers expressing high levels of HMGCoA reductase. J Cell Mol Med. 2010; 14:1180-93.

[76] Millatt LJ, Bocher V, Fruchart JC, Staels B. Liver X receptors and the control of cholesterol homeostasis: potential therapeutic targets for the treatment of atherosclerosis. Biochim Biophys Acta. 2003; 1631:107-18.

[77] Oosterveer MH, Grefhorst A, Groen AK, Kuipers F. The liver X receptor: control of cellular lipid homeostasis and beyond Implications for drug design. Prog Lipid Res. 2010; 49:343-52.

[78] Bovenga F, Sabbà C, Moschetta A. Uncoupling nuclear receptor LXR and cholesterol metabolism in cancer. Cell Metab. 2015; 21:517-26.

[79] Simon TG, Butt AA. Lipid dysregulation in hepatitis C virus, and impact of statin therapy upon clinical outcomes. World J Gastroenterol. 2015; 21:8293-303.

[80] Antoniou GA, Fisher RK, Georgiadis GS, Antoniou SA, Torella F. Statin therapy in lower limb peripheral arterial disease: systematic review and meta-analysis. Vascul Pharmacol. 2014; 63:79-87.

[81] Pang J, Chan DC, Watts GF. Critical review of non-statin treatments for dyslipoproteinemia. Expert Rev Cardiovasc Ther. 2014; 12:359-71.

[82] Szajnman SH, Ravaschino EL, Docampo R, Rodriguez JB. Synthesis and biological evaluation of 1-amino-1,1-bisphosphonates derived from fatty acids against Trypanosoma cruzi targeting farnesyl pyrophosphate synthase. Bioorg Med Chem Lett. 2005; 15:4685-90.

[83] Graaf MR, Richel DJ, van Noorden CJ, Guchelaar HJ. Effects of statins and farnesyltransferase inhibitors on the development and progression of cancer. Cancer Treat Rev. 2004; 30:609-41.

[84] Ugawa T, Kakuta H, Moritani H, Matsuda K, Ishihara T, Yamaguchi M, Naganuma S, Iizumi Y, Shikama H. YM-53601, a novel squalene synthase inhibitor, reduces plasma cholesterol and triglyceride levels in several animal species. Br J Pharmacol. 2000; 131:63-70.

[85] Nishimoto T, Ishikawa E, Anayama H, Hamajyo H, Nagai H, Hirakata M, Tozawa R. Protective effects of a squalene synthase inhibitor, lapaquistat acetate (TAK-475), on statin-induced myotoxicity in guinea pigs. Toxicol Appl Pharmacol. 2007; 223:39-45.

[86] Amin D, Rutledge RZ, Needle SN, Galczenski HF, Neuenschwander K, Scotese AC, Maguire MP, Bush RC, Hele DJ, Bilder GE, Perrone MH. RPR 107393, a potent squalene synthase inhibitor and orally effective cholesterol-lowering agent: comparison with inhibitors of HMG-CoA reductase. J Pharmacol Exp Ther. 1997; 281:746-52.

[87] Chuang JC, Valasek MA, Lopez AM, Posey KS, Repa JJ, Turley SD. Sustained and selective suppression of intestinal cholesterol synthesis by Ro 48-8071, an inhibitor of 2,3-oxidosqualene:lanosterol cyclase, in the BALB/c mouse. Biochem Pharmacol. 2014; 88:351-63.

[88] Eisele B, Budzinski R, Müller P, Maier R, Mark M. Effects of a novel 2,3-oxidosqualene cyclase inhibitor on cholesterol biosynthesis and lipid metabolism in vivo. J Lipid Res. 1997; 38:564-75.

[89] Ryder NS. Terbinafine: mode of action and properties of the squalene epoxidase inhibition. Br J Dermatol. 1992; 126 Suppl 39:2-7.

[90] Nutescu EA, Shapiro NL. Ezetimibe: a selective cholesterol absorption inhibitor. Pharmacotherapy. 2003; 23:1463-74.

[91] Lee M, Saver JL, Towfighi A, Chow J, Ovbiagele B. Efficacy of fibrates for cardiovascular risk reduction in persons with atherogenic dyslipidemia: a meta-analysis. Atherosclerosis. 2011; 217:492-8

[92] Wierzbicki AS. Fibrates: no ACCORD on their use in the treatment of dyslipidaemia. Curr Opin Lipidol. 2010; 21:352-8.

[93] Corsini A, Windler E, Farnier M. Colesevelam hydrochloride: usefulness of a specifically engineered bile acid sequestrant for lowering LDL-cholesterol. Eur J Cardiovasc Prev Rehabil. 2009; 16:1-9.

[94] Hou R, Goldberg AC. Lowering low-density lipoprotein cholesterol: statins, ezetimibe, bile acid sequestrants, and combinations: comparative efficacy and safety. Endocrinol Metab Clin North Am. 2009; 38:79-97.

[95] Llaverías G, Laguna JC, Alegret M. Pharmacology of the ACAT inhibitor avasimibe (CI-1011). Cardiovasc Drug Rev. 2003; 21:33-50.

[96] Koo SI, Noh SK. Green tea as inhibitor of the intestinal absorption of lipids: potential mechanism for its lipid-lowering effect. J Nutr Biochem. 2007; 18:179-83.

[97] Perry CM. Lomitapide: a review of its use in adults with homozygous familial hypercholesterolemia. Am J Cardiovasc Drugs. 2013; 13:285-96.

[98] Ricotta DN, Frishman W. Mipomersen: a safe and effective antisense therapy adjunct to statins in patients with hypercholesterolemia. Cardiol Rev. 2012; 20:90-5.

[99] Gutstein DE, Krishna R, Johns D, Surks HK, Dansky HM, Shah S, Mitchel YB, Arena J, Wagner JA. Anacetrapib, a novel CETP inhibitor: pursuing a new approach to cardiovascular risk reduction. Clin Pharmacol Ther. 2012; 91:109-22.

[100] Tavori H, Melone M, Rashid S. Alirocumab: PCSK9 inhibitor for LDL cholesterol reduction. Expert Rev Cardiovasc Ther. 2014; 12:1137-44.

[101] Cicero AF, Tartagni E, Ertek S. Efficacy and safety profile of evolocumab (AMG145), an injectable inhibitor of the proprotein convertase subtilisin/kexin type 9: the available clinical evidence. Expert Opin Biol Ther. 2014; 14:863-8.

[102] Preta G, Cronin JG, Sheldon IM. Dynasore - not just a dynamin inhibitor. Cell Commun Signal. 2015; 13:24.

[103] Gbelcová H, Lenícek M, Zelenka J, Knejzlík Z, Dvoráková G, Zadinová M, Poucková P, Kudla M, Balaz P, Ruml T, Vítek L. Differences in antitumor effects of various statins on human pancreatic cancer. Int J Cancer. 2008; 122:1214-21.

[104] Benakanakere I, Johnson T, Sleightholm R, Villeda V, Arya M, Bobba R, Freter C, Huang C. Targeting cholesterol synthesis increases chemoimmuno-sensitivity in chronic lymphocytic leukemia cells. Exp Hematol Oncol. 2014; 3:24.

[105] Lin CJ, Liao WC, Lin HJ, Hsu YM, Lin CL, Chen YA, Feng CL, Chen CJ, Kao MC, Lai CH, Kao CH. Statins attenuate Helicobacter pylori CagA translocation and reduce incidence of gastric cancer: in vitro and population-based case-control studies. PLoS One. 2016; 11:e0146432.

[106] Bjarnadottir O, Romero Q, Bendahl PO, Jirström K, Rydén L, Loman N, Uhlén M, Johannesson H, Rose C, Grabau D, Borgquist S. Targeting HMG-CoA reductase with statins in a window-of-opportunity breast cancer trial. Breast Cancer Res Treat. 2013; 138:499-508.

[107] Sehdev A, O'Neil BH. The role of aspirin, vitamin D, exercise, diet, statins, and metformin in the prevention and treatment of colorectal cancer. Curr Treat Opt Oncol. 2015; 16:43.

[108] Peng YC, Lin CL, Hsu WY, Chang CS, Yeh HZ, Tung CF, Wu YL, Sung FC, Kao CH. Statins are associated with a reduced risk of cholangiocarcinoma: a population-based case-control study. Br J Clin Pharmacol. 2015; 80:755-61.

[109] Jacobs EJ, Rodriguez C, Bain EB, Wang Y, Thun MJ, Calle EE. Cholesterol-lowering drugs and advanced prostate cancer incidence in a large U.S. cohort. Cancer Epidemiol Biomark Prev. 2007; 16:2213-7.

[110] Vinogradova Y, Hippisley-Cox J, Coupland C, Logan RF. Risk of colorectal cancer in patients prescribed statins, nonsteroidal anti-inflammatory drugs, and cyclooxygenase-2 inhibitors: nested case-control study. Gastroenterology. 2007; 133:393-402.

[111] Jacobs EJ, Rodriguez C, Brady KA, Connell CJ, Thun MJ, Calle EE. Cholesterol-lowering drugs and colorectal cancer incidence in a large United States cohort. J Natl Cancer Inst. 2006; 98:69-72.

[112] Raval AD, Thakker D, Negi H, Vyas A, Salkini MW. Association between statins and clinical outcomes among men with prostate cancer: a systematic review and meta-analysis. Prostate Cancer Prostatic Dis. 2016; doi: 10.1038/pcan.2015.58.

[113] McKay RR, Lin X, Albiges L, Fay AP, Kaymakcalan MD, Mickey SS, Ghoroghchian PP, Bhatt RS, Kaffenberger SD, Simantov R, Choueiri TK, Heng DY. Statins and survival outcomes in patients with metastatic renal cell carcinoma. Eur J Cancer. 2016; 52:155-62.

[114] Freeman SR, Drake AL, Heilig LF, Graber M, McNealy K, Schilling LM, Dellavalle RP. Statins, fibrates, and melanoma risk: a systematic review and meta-analysis. J Natl Cancer Inst. 2006; 98:1538-46.

[115] Hwa JJ, Zollman S, Warden CH, Taylor BA, Edwards PA, Fogelman AM, Lusis AJ. Genetic and dietary interactions in the regulation of HMG-CoA reductase gene expression. J Lipid Res. 1992; 33:711-25.

[116] Horton JD, Goldstein JL, Brown MS. SREBPs: activators of the complete program of cholesterol and fatty acid synthesis in the liver. J Clin Invest 2002; 109:1125–31.

[117] Wu N, Sarna LK, Hwang SY, Zhu Q, Wang P, Siow YL, O K. Activation of 3-hydroxy-3-methylglutaryl coenzyme A (HMG-CoA) reductase during high fat diet feeding. Biochim Biophys Acta. 2013; 1832:1560-8.

[118] Martínez-Botas J, Suárez Y, Ferruelo AJ, Gómez-Coronado D, Lasuncion MA. Cholesterol starvation decreases p34(cdc2) kinase activity and arrests the cell cycle at G2. FASEB J. 1999; 13:1359-70.

[119] Tsubaki M, Yamazoe Y, Yanae M, Satou T, Itoh T, Kaneko J, Kidera Y, Moriyama K, Nishida S. Blockade of the Ras/MEK/ERK and Ras/PI3K/Akt pathways by statins reduces the expression of bFGF, HGF, and TGF-β as angiogenic factors in mouse osteosarcoma. Cytokine. 2011; 54:100-7.

[120] Zhu Y, Casey PJ, Kumar AP, Pervaiz S. Deciphering the signaling networks underlying simvastatin-induced apoptosis in human cancer cells: evidence for non-canonical activation of RhoA and Rac1 GTPases. Cell Death Dis 2013; 4:e568.

[121] Woodard J, Sassano A, Hay N, Platanias LC. Statin-dependent suppression of the Akt/mammalian target of rapamycin signaling cascade and programmed cell death 4 up-regulation in renal cell carcinoma. Clin Cancer Res 2008; 14:4640-4649.

[122] Weis M, Heeschen C, Glassford AJ, Cooke JP. Statins have biphasic effects on angiogenesis. Circulation. 2002; 105:739-45.

[123] Kidera Y, Tsubaki M, Yamazoe Y, Shoji K, Nakamura H, Ogaki M, Satou T, Itoh T, Isozaki M, Kaneko J, Tanimori Y, Yanae M, Nishida S. Reduction of lung metastasis, cell invasion, and adhesion in mouse melanoma by statin-induced blockade of the Rho/Rho-associated coiled-coil-containing protein kinase pathway. J Exp Clin Cancer Res. 2010; 29:127.

[124] Murai T. The role of lipid rafts in cancer cell adhesion and migration. Int J Cell Biol. 2012; 2012:763283.

[125] Jeon JH, Kim SK, Kim HJ, Chang J, Ahn CM, Chang YS. Lipid raft modulation inhibits NSCLC cell migration through delocalization of the focal adhesion complex. Lung Cancer. 2010; 69:165-71.

[126] Coleman PS. Membrane cholesterol and tumor bioenergetics. Ann N Y Acad Sci. 1986; 488:451-67.

[127] Swyer G. The cholesterol content of normal and enlarged prostates. Cancer Res 1942; 2:372–375.

[128] Singer SJ, Nicolson GL. The fluid mosaic model of the structure of cell membranes. Science 1972; 175:720-731.

[129] Bonovas S, Filioussi K, Sitaras NM. Statins are not associated with a reduced risk of pancreatic cancer at the population level, when taken at low doses for managing hypercholesterolemia: evidence from a meta-analysis of 12 studies. Am J Gastroenterol. 2008; 103:2646-51.

[130] Khurana V, Sheth A, Caldito G, Barkin JS. Statins reduce the risk of pancreatic cancer in humans: a case-control study of half a million veterans. Pancreas. 2007; 34:260-5.

[131] Singh PP, Singh S. Statins are associated with reduced risk of gastric cancer: a systematic review and meta-analysis. Ann Oncol. 2013; 24:1721-30.

[132] Tsan YT, Lee CH, Wang JD, Chen PC. Statins and the risk of hepatocellular carcinoma in patients with hepatitis B virus infection. J Clin Oncol. 2012; 30:623-30.

[133] Chen HH, Lin MC, Muo CH, Yeh SY, Sung FC, Kao CH. Combination therapy of metformin and statin may decrease hepatocellular carcinoma among diabetic patients in Asia. Medicine (Baltimore). 2015; 94:e1013.

[134] Zhang XL, Geng J, Zhang XP, Peng B, Che JP, Yan Y, Wang GC, Xia SQ, Wu Y, Zheng JH. Statin use and risk of bladder cancer: a meta-analysis. Cancer Causes Control. 2013; 24:769-76.

[135] Yi X, Jia W, Jin Y, Zhen S. Statin use is associated with reduced risk of haematological malignancies: evidence from a meta-analysis. PLoS One. 2014; 9:e87019.

[136] Pradelli D, Soranna D, Zambon A, Catapano A, Mancia G, La Vecchia C, Corrao G. Statins use and the risk of all and subtype hematological malignancies: a meta-analysis of observational studies. Cancer Med. 2015;4(5):770-80.

[137] Wang J, Li C, Tao H, Cheng Y, Han L, Li X, Hu Y. Statin use and risk of lung cancer: a meta-analysis of observational studies and randomized controlled trials. PLoS One. 2013; 8:e77950.

[138] Bansal D, Undela K, D'Cruz S, Schifano F. Statin use and risk of prostate cancer: a meta-analysis of observational studies. PLoS One. 2012; 7:e46691.

[139] Undela K, Srikanth V, Bansal D. Statin use and risk of breast cancer: a meta-analysis of observational studies. Breast Cancer Res Treat. 2012; 135:261-9.

[140] Lytras T, Nikolopoulos G, Bonovas S. Statins and the risk of colorectal cancer: an updated systematic review and meta-analysis of 40 studies. World J Gastroenterol. 2014; 20:1858-70.

[141] Setoguchi S, Glynn RJ, Avorn J, Mogun H, Schneeweiss S. Statins and the risk of lung, breast, and colorectal cancer in the elderly. Circulation. 2007; 115:27-33.

[142] Kuoppala J, Lamminpää A, Pukkala E. Statins and cancer: a systematic review and meta-analysis. Eur J Cancer. 2008; 44:2122-32.

[143] Song C, Park S, Park J, Shim M, Kim A, Jeong IG, Hong JH, Kim CS, Ahn H. Statin use after radical prostatectomy reduces biochemical recurrence in men with prostate cancer. Prostate. 2015; 75:211-7.

[144] Cai H, Zhang G, Wang Z, Luo Z, Zhou X. Relationship between the use of statins and patient survival in colorectal cancer: a systematic review and meta-analysis. PLoS One. 2015; 10:e0126944.

[145] Cardwell CR, Hicks BM, Hughes C, Murray LJ. Statin use after colorectal cancer diagnosis and survival: a population-based cohort study. J Clin Oncol. 2014; 32:3177-83.

[146] Kozak MM, Anderson EM, von Eyben R, Pai JS, Poultsides GA, Visser BC, Norton JA, Koong AC, Chang DT. Statin and metformin use prolongs survival in patients with resectable pancreatic cancer. Pancreas. 2016; 45:64-70.

[147] Jeon CY, Pandol SJ, Wu B, Cook-Wiens G, Gottlieb RA, Merz CN, Goodman MT. The association of statin use after cancer diagnosis with survival in pancreatic cancer patients: a SEER-medicare analysis. PLoS One. 2015; 10:e0121783.

[148] Wu BU, Chang J, Jeon CY, Pandol SJ, Huang B, Ngor EW, Difronzo AL, Cooper RM. Impact of statin use on survival in patients undergoing resection for early-stage pancreatic cancer. Am J Gastroenterol. 2015; 110:1233-9.

[149] Lacerda L, Reddy JP, Liu D, Larson R, Li L, Masuda H, Brewer T, Debeb BG, Xu W, Hortobágyi GN, Buchholz TA, Ueno NT, Woodward WA. Simvastatin radiosensitizes differentiated and stem-like breast cancer cell lines and is associated with improved local control in inflammatory breast cancer patients treated with postmastectomy radiation. Stem Cells Transl Med. 2014; 3:849-56.

[150] Winiarska M, Bil J, Wilczek E, Wilczynski GM, Lekka M, Engelberts PJ, Mackus WJ, Gorska E, Bojarski L, Stoklosa T, Nowis D, Kurzaj Z, Makowski M, Glodkowska E, Issat T, Mrowka P, Lasek W, Dabrowska-Iwanicka A, Basak GW, Wasik M, Warzocha K, Sinski M, Gaciong Z, Jakobisiak M, Parren PW, Golab J. Statins impair antitumor effects of rituximab by inducing conformational changes of CD20. PLoS Med. 2008; 5:e64.

[151] Hoffmeister M, Jansen L, Rudolph A, Toth C, Kloor M, Roth W, Bläker H, Chang-Claude J, Brenner H. Statin use and survival after colorectal cancer: the importance of comprehensive confounder adjustment. J Natl Cancer Inst. 2015; 107:djv045.

Chapter 7

Ethnicity and Response to Drug Therapy

Maha M. Alrasheed and Nduna Dzimiri

Additional information is available at the end of the chapter

http://dx.doi.org/10.5772/64819

Abstract

Hypercholesterolemia is a complex disorder presenting in different forms, including the familial form (FH), with varying underlying aetiology, and contributing substantially to coronary artery disease. Particularly, the FH underlies monogenic changes in genes involved in cholesterol synthesis and transport, including the low density lipoprotein receptor, proprotein convertase sublitisin/kexin type 9 and apolipoprotein B. However, hyperlipidemia is largely a complex interaction of changes in multiple genes with environmental factors, such as diet, overweight and obesity that are controllable by adopting healthy eating habits and exercise, which may vary by ethnicity. Diet alone is often not adequate to achieve the desired lipid lowering effect in individuals harbouring very high cholesterol levels, necessitating the use of lipid lowering medication or other forms of therapy. Antilipidemic drugs fall into (a) bile acid sequestrants (b) cholesterol absorption inhibitors, (c) 3-hydroxy-3-methylglutaryl coenzyme A reductase inhibitors, (d) fibric acid derivatives (e) proprotein convertase subtilisin/kexin type 9 inhibitors, (f) miscellaneous agents and (g) drug combinations. Mutations in their various metabolizing enzymes, particularly the cytochrome P450 family, often lead to partially/non-functional, or even rapid metabolizing phenotypes, triggering great variations in the way individuals respond to drug therapy, which in turn depends on ethnicity. This may produce unexpected outcomes such as therapeutic failure, adverse side effects and toxicity in individuals of different ethnic origin. Hence, in-depth information of the impact of ethnicity on these relationships has the huge potential of achieving optimal quality use of drugs as well as improving the efficacy and safety of antilipidemic therapeutic agents.

Keywords: cholesterol, hypercholesterolemia, ethnicity, gene polymorphism, polygenic complex disease, anti-lipidemic drug therapy, drug metabolism

1. Introduction

Cholesterol is a sterol that presents one of the three major classes of lipids synthesized and utilized by animal cells to construct their cell membranes. It also serves as a precursor of the steroid hormones, bile acids and vitamin D, and is transported in the blood plasma within lipoproteins. These lipoproteins are classified according to their density as (a) very-low-density lipoproteins (VLDLs), (b) low-density lipoproteins (LDLs), (c) intermediate-density lipoproteins (IDLs) and (d) high-density lipoproteins (HDLs) [1]. Hypercholesterolemia (also often referred to as dyslipidemia) describes a condition characterized by elevated lipid (hyperlipidemia) or lipoprotein levels (hyperlipoproteinemia) (>240 mg/dL) in circulation [2]. Such elevated levels of lipoproteins, other than HDL (also called non-HDL-cholesterol), particularly the LDL-cholesterol, are associated with an increased risk of coronary artery disease (CAD) [3]. In contrast, increased HDL-cholesterol levels are deemed protective [4]. An elevation in circulating non-HDL- and LDL-cholesterol may be triggered by diet, obesity, genetic disorders or presence of other diseases, such as diabetes and dysfunctional thyroid [2, 5]. Hyperlipidemia is one of the most important players in developing cardiovascular disease leading to high mortality [6, 7]. Hence, management of hyperlipidemia not only maintains healthy lipoprotein levels, but is also designed to avert the more deleterious consequences of CAD manifestation.

Hyperlipidemia affects humans globally with a prevalence of approximate 34 million in the USA. It occurs partly as an inheritable monogenic (Mendelian) disease, specifically the familial form, which affects 1 in 500 individuals globally, but more frequently so, as a result of an interaction of genetic changes with environmental factors, that may or may not be modifiable. Inheritable forms include the familial types, such as homozygous familial hypercholesterolemia (HOFH) or familial hyperbetalipoproteinemia (FHBL), a disorder that impairs the body's capability to absorb and transport fats. This form of the disease is characterized by early signs of cholesterol infiltrates with premature CAD, accompanied by a building up of excess cholesterol in other tissues such as the skin, tendons and coronary arteries. This, in turn, is also accompanied by growths defined as tendon xanthomas, known to affect the Achilles tendons as well as tendons in hands and fingers [8]. Other forms of cholesterol deposits also exist, such as xanthelasmata under the eyelid skin and cornealis, accumulating at the edge of the clear front surface of the cornea. The complex form of hypercholesterolemia is triggered by some interplay between genetic variants with modifiable risk factors, such as lifestyle or diet and/or unmodifiable variables, such as age, ethnicity, gender and family history. Some of the modifiable predisposing factors such as diet, overweight and obesity are controllable by adopting a healthy eating plan, staying active and managing personal weight scale. However, patients with very high cholesterol levels, such as in familial hypercholesterolemia (FH), diet alone is often not adequate to achieve the desired lipid lowering effect, necessitating the use of lipid lowering medication to reduce its production and absorption [9], as well as other therapies including LDL apheresis or surgery. Several drug families are employed targeting different components of cholesterol metabolism. The success of treatment may vary in different communities, depending on a number of contributing factors, particularly ethnicity. Importantly, while the influence of the unmodifiable risk traits is likely to be felt alike across ethnicities, their actual impact on disease will often be defined by the extent to which genetic changes interact with these environmental factors within a given population. These risk factors can also influence drug response and toxicity, whereby the penetrance of these interactions on disease and drug therapeutic outcomes similarly depends on ethnicity, with some influence of the confounding modifiable risk factors. This chapter therefore focuses on the impact of ethnicity on interaction of these predisposing factors, particular genetic polymorphism, in the management of hypercholesterolemia.

2. Ethnicity and hypercholesterolemia

Blood lipid levels are highly heritable traits. Essentially, hypercholesterolemia occurs as a result of the low-density lipoprotein receptor (LDLR) being unable to remove cholesterol effectively from circulation. This can be caused by mutations in one or more genes that regulate cholesterol metabolism and transportation. The greatest contribution to the manifestation of hypercholesterolemia and difficulties related to maintaining health circulating cholesterol levels are genetic changes in components of these pathways. While only a handful of Mendelian disease genes and founder mutations for the autosomal recessive form of the disease have been identified to date, there are many other genes that contribute to the complex form of the disease. Thus, whereas the Mendelian form is likely to exert the same impact globally, the manifestation of the complex trait will more often than not depend on the nature of the interactions between the predisposing genes and environmental factors, which may vary among various ethnicities. This, in turn, has a great impact on disease manifestation in a given society.

2.1. Ethnicity, race ancestry and disease

Ethnicity and race have traditionally been related to biological and sociological factors, respectively. Accordingly, race presumes shared biological or genetic traits and is distinguishable by the traits resulting from a shared genealogy due to geographical demarcations, while ethnicity connotes shared cultural traits and history, and possibly linguistic or religious traits. In terms of genetic undertones, therefore, individuals of the same racial background (ancestry) are likely to carry more common genetic architecture than those belonging to the same ethnicity. Hence, the impact of these two societal confounders on dyslipidemia manifestation may not always be the same. Besides, in multi-cultural societies, such as in the USA or Southern Africa, many (ethnic) admixture groups have arisen in the course of time, from different ancestral lineage, and are often placed into the one or the other ethnical group. This adds some complexity to the estimation of the depth of genetic adulteration in racial genetic texture, rendering the ancestral delineation more complex. Accordingly, the impact of intra-ethnical variations on disease might be over- or underestimated within a given community. Most importantly, the influence of ethnicity on the disease manifestation or therapeutic outcome is also often regulated by modifiable confounders as well as the depth of public awareness within a given society. Hence, the accuracy in the estimation of the depth of the influence of ethnicity on dyslipidemia and therapy thereof may depend on the constituent racial component of the given society.

2.2. Ethnicity and genetics of hypercholesterolemia

Genetically, hypercholesterolemia may occur in various forms depending on the type and genomic location of the causative mutation. This may directly be caused by a structural change in a gene involved in the transportation of the lipids. Thus, the monogenic (Mendelian) form, often manifest as familial hypercholesterolemia (FH), is triggered by changes in a single gene. To date, the monogenic form has been linked primarily to mutations in three genes, the LDLR [10–15], proprotein convertase sublitisin/kexin type 9 (PCSK9) [16–23] and apolipoprotein B (APOB) genes [24–28]. In most cases, individuals with FH will have inherited one or both altered copies of the gene from affected parents. In this case, the disease can be acquired in an autosomal recessive (presence of two copies of the mutated gene from both parents) such as the autosomal recessive hypercholesterolemia (ARH), or in a dominant (presence of only one copy of the mutated gene from either parent) form such as HOFH or heterozygous familial disease (HEFH). The recessive type tends to lead to the more severe form of the disease, which often appears in childhood. The HEFH is a very rare form of FH, affecting a small but noticeable percentage of individuals, yet constituting an important cause of early onset of CAD. The disease results from either biallelic pathogenic variants in one of the three genes or one pathogenic variant in each of two different genes. It is thought to account for 60–80% of FH.

However, the most common forms of hyperlipidemia are complex in nature, resulting primarily from an interaction between genetic changes and environmental factors [29]. Thus, apart from the three genes, *LDLR*, *APOB* and *PCSK9*, known to cause the monogenic disease, several others are also involved in the manifestation of the disease. The genes include the peroxisome proliferator-activated receptor-alpha (*PPAR-α*), cholesteryl ester transport protein (*CETP*), low-density lipoprotein receptor adaptor protein 1 (*LDLRAP1*), apolipoprotein (APO) A1 (APOA1), A4 and A5 complex (*APOA1/A4/A5*) and apolipoprotein E (*APOE*), 3-hyroxy-3-methylglutaryl coenzyme A reductase (HMGR), lecithin cholesterolacyltransferase (LCAT) and lipoprotein lipase (LPL), just to name a few. The genes associated with the different forms of dyslipidemia are summarized in **Table 1**.

Among the genes associated with dyslipidemia to date, the *LDLR* is understandably the most well defined. This gene encodes the LDLR protein which binds to low-density lipoproteins (LDLs) particles, the primary carriers of cholesterol in the blood. This receptor resides on the outer surface of many cell types, particularly in the liver, where it picks up circulating LDL particles and transports them into the cell. Within the cell, the receptor is broken down in order to release cholesterol for utilization by the cell, storage or removal from the body. The LDLR is essential in regulating the amount of circulating cholesterol, whereby the speed at which the later gets eliminated from the system depends on the receptor expression. Hence, alteration in the structure of these receptors will lead to fundamental changes in the regulation of circulating cholesterol levels. Such mutations in the *LDLR* gene are thought to be the primary cause for FH, with a greater frequency in a population with founder mutations. Several such hyperlipidemia-related variants have been identified thus far in this gene [10–15]. These mutations have different effects on the function of the protein. For example, some of them do so by reducing the number of LDLRs produced within the cells, while others disrupt the ability of the receptors to remove the LDLs from circulation. As a result, individuals harbouring *LDLR* mutations will have very high circulating cholesterol levels, ultimately leading to the familial form of the disease. Some of these mutations have been implicated in both the autosomal recessive (ARH) and dominant (ADH) forms of hypercholesterolemia, whereby in some ethnic populations, the ADH has been shown to exhibit allelic heterogeneity [11, 30]. Thus, genetic diversity has been described in FH [30, 31], pointing to the likelihood of differences in the extent to which these mutations may cause disease in different populations. This may be ascribable to differences in life style. It has also been suggested that the *LDLR* gene has a sex-specific pleiotropic effect, as is indicated by changes in the relationship between traits [32]. This suggests in turn that environmental factors, such as diet or even migration, may play a significant role in modulating the phenotype of heterozygous FH.

Gene	**Chr locus**	**Protein function**	**Mechanism**	**Disorder (mutations)**
APO A1	11q23.3	Promotes Chol efflux from tissue to the liver for excretion.	Cofactor for LCAT	hTG; HDL deficiencies; Tangier disease; HALP
APO A4	11q23.3	Major HDL and chylomicron component; chylomicron and VLDL secretion and catabolism	Required for lipoprotein lipase activation by ApoC-II; potent activator of LCAT	Chronic inflammatory demyelinating polyneuropathy
APO A5	11q23.3	Regulating plasma TG levels; inhibitor of hepatic VLDL production	Minor apolipoprotein associated with HDL, may activates LCAT	hTG; HLP
APOB	2p24-p23	Internalization of LDL particles by apoB receptor	Recognition signal for cellular binding; major constituent of LDL and VLDL	FHBL (>50); HL; FDB (>5), ADH
APOE	19q13.2	Ligand for LDLR and specific apo-E receptor (chylomicron remnant) of hepatic tissues	Mediates binding, internalization and catabolism of lipoprotein particles	Polygenic HL; HLP type II and III
CETP	16q21	Transfer of neutral lipids, e.g. cholesteryl ester and triglyceride among lipoprotein particles	Allows net movement of choles teryl ester from HDL to TG-rich VLDL and TG and vice versa	HALP; hTG, Low HDLC
LDLR	19p13.2	Intracellular cholesterol transfer and transport in blood	Binding to bile acids in intestines	FH (>1000)
LDLRAP1	1p36.11	LDL binding and internalization; endocytosis	Adapter protein for LDLR endocytosis in hepatocytes and lymphocytes	HL (>10)
PCSK9	1p32.3	Regulation cholesterol homeostasis	Binds to LDLRs, VLDLR, APOER, APOER2	Familial HBLP
PPAR-α	3p25.2	Key regulator of lipid metabolism	Binds to peroxisome proliferators, e.g. hypolipidemic drugs	

ADH, autosomal dominant hypercholesterolemia; ApoB, apolipoprotein B; APOER, apolipoprotein receptor; CETP, cholesteryl ester transport protein; FDB, familial defective apoB-100; Chol, cholesterol; Chr; chromosomal position; FH, familial hypercholesterolemia; FHBL, familial hyperbetalipoproteinemia; HALP, hypoalphalipoproteinemia; HBLP, hypobetalipoproteinemia; HDLC, high-density lipoprotein-cholesterol; HMG-CoA; 3-hyroxy-3-methylglutaryl coenzyme A reductase; HLP, hyperlipoproteinemia; hTG, hypertriglyceridemia; LCAT, lecithin cholesterol acyltransferase; LDLR, low-density lipoprotein receptor; LDLRAP1, low-density lipoprotein receptor adaptor protein 1; LPL, lipoprotein; PCSK9, proprotein convertase sublitisin/kexin type 9; PPAR-α, peroxisome proliferator-activated receptor-alpha; VLDL, very-low-density lipoprotein.

Table 1. Gene polymorphisms currently known to contribute to hypercholesterolemia.

One other important gene involved in HL is that encoding the apolipoprotein B (apoB) proteins. This gene encodes two versions of the protein: a shorter version (apoB-48) and a longer version (apoB-100). Both isoforms are involved in transporting fat-like particles, including cholesterol, in the blood. They are synthesized primarily in two organs, whereby the apoB-48 is produced in the intestines, while the apoB-100 is synthesized primarily in the liver. The former functions as a component of the chylomicron lipoproteins and is important for the absorption of certain fat-soluble vitamins, such as the vitamins A and E. The apoB-100, on the other hand, constitutes a component of other forms of lipoproteins, specifically the VLDLs, IDLs and LDLs, all of which are involved in the transportation of fats and cholesterol in the blood. Accordingly, apoB facilitates the LDL binding to their receptors in the liver cell surface. This in turn enables the transportation of these lipoproteins into the cell, where they are broken down to facilitate the release of cholesterol. Thus, mutations in the *APOB* gene can cause familial hyperbetalipoproteinemia (FHBL) or hypercholesterolemia by triggering the production of abnormally short forms of the protein, and therefore a reduction or lack of dietary fat and cholesterol transportation and ultimately the body's ability to absorb fats and fat-soluble vitamins from the diet. The severity of the disease depends on the length of the abnormal protein. Accordingly, a resultant protein that is longer than the apoB-48 will not hamper its production; hence, it should still be capable of forming chylomicrons. On the other hand, a similar product of the apoB-100 in the liver will not be able to produce LPLs efficiently. Hence, protein products that are shorter than the apoB are associated with more severe symptoms than in cases where some normal apoB-48 is produced. *APOB* mutations may also trigger the familial ligand-defective apoB-100 (FDB) [27] and ADH conditions [26]. These states are characterized by the presence of very high circulating cholesterol levels and therefore increased risk of disease. The impact of genetic changes in *APOB* on hypercholesterolemia is, however, less described than that of the *LDLR* gene. Besides, there has been some inconsistences in reports on the impact of some of these mutations in different populations [10], pointing to its variation by ethnicity [33, 34].

The proprotein convertase sublitisin/kexin type 9 (PCSK9) functions by enhancing the regulation of circulating cholesterol levels, thereby possibly controlling the number of LDLRs on the cell surface. It probably acts by breaking down the LDLRs before they reach the cell surface. A few hypercholesterolemia-related mutations have been reported in the PCSK9 to date [16, 35], and have been linked mainly to ADH [20–23]. Accordingly, the mutations responsible for the disease are termed 'gain-of-function' mutations as they enhance the protein activity or lead to the protein acquiring new atypical functions. Serum lipoprotein Lp(a) is thought to be elevated in FH as a result of such PCSK9 gain-of-function mutations [18, 19], for example. The overactive protein significantly reduces the number of LDLRs on the surface of the liver cells, possibly by triggering faster breakage of the LDLRs. Thus, the attenuated production of the receptors leads to more cholesterol accumulation, and therefore the possibility of the disease occurring. Other mutations in the gene defined as 'loss-of-function' mutations reduce blood cholesterol levels (hypocholesterolemia) by decreasing the PSCK9 activity or reducing its amount in the cell. These mutations lead to an increase in the number of LDLRs on the surface of liver cells. Harbouring of such mutation has been linked to a significantly lower than average risk of developing heart disease. Furthermore, elevated

PCSK9 levels are thought to be detrimental for patients carrying either non-FH or HEFH [36], since they tend to correlate with LDL-cholesterol levels [37].

The PPAR-α, $-\beta/\gamma$ are ligand-activated transcription factors serving as the primary regulators of several activities including glucose, fatty acid and lipoprotein metabolism, energy balance, cell proliferation and differentiation, inflammation and atherosclerosis. Thereby, the PPAR-α activates the lipoprotein lipase (LPL) to ultimately reduce the formation of VLDL-cholesterol and triglycerides as well as increasing HDL-cholesterol. The genes have been collectively implicated in hypertriglyceridemia [38], possibly through gene-gene interactive mechanisms, and may modulate the risk of CAD by influencing both fasting and postprandial lipid concentrations [39]. Together with the PPAR-γ, the PPAR-α has also been implicated in HL [40–43] and low HDL levels [44, 45].

As the name denotes, the function of cholesteryl ester transfer protein (CETP) is to transfer neutral lipids, such as cholesteryl ester, forming cholesterol among lipoprotein particles. Specifically, it controls the net influx of cholesteryl ester from HDL to triglyceride-rich VLDL and the equimolar transport of triglyceride from VLDL to HDL. Thus, it regulates the reverse cholesterol transport through which the lipid is removed from peripheral tissue and returned to the liver for elimination. Defects such as *CETP Taq1B* polymorphism in the encoding gene have been implicated in harbouring of low HDL-cholesterol [46, 47] and hypertriglyceridemia [48].

The low-density lipoprotein receptor adaptor protein 1 (*LDLRAP1*) acts essentially by influencing the function of the LDLRs. Hence, mutations in this gene would either prevent the cell from making functional receptors or alter their function. It probably interacts with the LDLRs thereby removing them together with the attached LDLs from the cell surface to the interior of the cell to facilitate the breaking down of the latter and the release of cholesterol. In the absence of a functional LDLRA1 protein, LDLR particles cannot be transported into the cell, even if they bind normally to them. This triggers the retention of the lipids in circulation, therefore leading to abnormally high cholesterol levels. Mutations in the gene have been associated with ARH [49–52]. This is thought to be a result of the gene producing an abnormally small, non-functional version of the protein or preventing the cell from making the functional protein.

The apolipoprotein A-1 promotes cholesterol efflux from tissue to the liver for excretion. It is also a co-factor for lecithin cholesterol acyltransferase (LCAT), which is responsible for the formation of the majority of cholesteryl esters. Some recent reports indicate that the increase in HDL-cholesterol on statin treatment may also be influenced by *APOA1* genotypes. The *APOA1* gene is closely linked to three other apolipoprotein genes, *APOA4*, *APOA5* and *APOC3* in a cluster form of *APOA1/C3/A4/A5* on chromosome 11. This complex has been associated with hypertriglyceridemia in various ethnic groups [53, 54]. The *APOA4* gene is a major component of HDL and chylomicrons, but not so much associated with VLDL. It is thought to be a potent activator of LCAT. It may play a role in chylomicrons and VLDL secretion and catabolism, and is needed by the apoC-II for efficient activation of LPL. The apo A5 regulates plasma triglyceride levels by acting both as a potent stimulator of triglyceride hydrolysis by apoC II-mediated LPL activity and as an inhibitor of hepatic VLDL production. However, its activation of LCAT is weak and does not enhance the efflux of cholesterol from macrophages. The *APOA5* gene polymorphism has been associated with hypertriglyceridemia and hyperlipoproteinemia type 5 [54].

The apolipoprotein E (*APOE*) polymorphism is regulated through three common alleles, epsilon 2, 3 and 4, coding for proteins that differ in lipoprotein receptor binding activity or their catabolism. This lipoprotein contains two different polypeptides apoB-100 and the (lipoprotein) Lp(a) glycoprotein. The latter exhibits a genetic polymorphism that is regulated by a series of autosomal alleles at a single locus and is associated with lipoprotein plasma concentrations. This suggests that the same gene locus is involved in determining Lp(a) glycoprotein phenotypes and its plasma concentrations. Hence, variability in apolipoprotein genes related to the normal variance of lipoprotein concentrations play a major genetic role in multi-factorial forms of HL such as hTG, familial type III HL, polygenic HL [55] and ADH [24].

Although FH is thought to be monogenic to a greater part, some inter-ethnical differences have been reported in the prevalence of the disease. In the USA, for example, dyslipidemia is thought to be highly prevalent among Hispanics (Latinos), with Cubans appearing to be particularly at risk, possibly explained by socio-economic status and acculturation [56], while increased African ancestry has been apparently linked to a decrease in triglyceride and LDLC as well as increased HDLC levels [57]. Also, lower odds for combined hyperlipidemia have been demonstrated for African-Americans compared to whites, despite higher body mass index (BMI) and abnormal adiposity, while Hispanics had slightly higher and Asian no difference odds to whites [58]. These differences may to a greater part be due to variations in the genetic modifiers among ethnic groups, a subject that continues to be unravelled. Similarly, the prevalence of the CEPT polymorphism appears to vary among ethnic groups as suggested by a Singaporean study reporting highest prevalence in Indian and lowest in the Malays with the Chinese showing an intermediate value, while African-American veterans exhibited higher blood pressure, LDL-cholesterol and protein A1c levels than Whites [59]. Differences have also been reported in the distribution of the *APOA5* gene variants in various ethnic groups in China [54] and Singapore [59]. These variations have been partly linked to the existence of population admixture [60]. It has also been observed that some polymorphic gene locus controls the concentrations of Lp(a) lipoprotein complex in plasma which may vary very widely between individuals. Hence, variability in apolipoprotein genes related to the normal variance of lipoprotein concentrations play a major genetic role in multi-factorial forms of HL such as hTG, familial type III HL and polygenic HL [55], as well as ADH [24]. Furthermore, the effects of the *APOE* alleles on the phenotypic variance of plasma lipoprotein concentrations have been found to differ significantly among ethnic groups. This has been explained by the fact that APOE polymorphism encodes different proteins with different binding properties. However, to date, most of the large-scale studies have been performed primarily in individuals of European descent, but many other ethnic groups have not been exhaustively studied yet. Importantly, due to lack of studies in such populations, we might be missing important data relevant in the influence of ethnicity of the manifestation of the disease. For example, it is quite likely that because of consanguinity among ethnic Arab populations, their prevalence would rank among the highest in the world. Therefore, data needs to be collected on such populations to define more precisely the impact of ethnicity on the relationship between gene polymorphism and HL manifestation, which is likely to be unique for that particular ethnic group. Nonetheless, these data furnish support to the notion of the inter-ethnic variations in lipid traits being linked to genetic variants that exhibit differences in frequencies in individuals of African, Asian and European ancestry [61]. Besides, differences in lifestyle, such as leisure time, smoking and pedantic life style, for example, will also exert an impact on the disease manifestation, as demonstrated by the different levels of awareness of health risks among urban population compared to rural ones. Therefore, their ultimate effect on disease manifestation may vary between different ethnic groups, even within a given society.

2.3. Confounders for ethnicity interactions with hyperlipidemia disease

As stated above, in the majority of cases, HL is a product of an interaction of a combination of lifestyle choices with structural alterations in a multiple of genes, rather than a result of a single inherited condition. The disease penetrance will be dependent on the prevalence of various risk factors, including diet, exercise and tobacco smoking, but more importantly gender and age. The latter are also important determinants of the influence of dyslipidemia and other diseases, such as diabetes and obesity, on the manifestation of CAD. Ultimately, the impact of these interactions on dyslipidemia varies by ethnicity. The impact of ethnicity on HL manifestation is, in turn, also greatly influenced by these lifestyle confounders, particularly the modifiable variables, such as obesity, diet and lifestyle. According to the World Health Organisation (WHO), obesity is a condition in which the body accumulates fat to the extent that the health and well-being of the individual are adversely affected [62]. The primary causes for this disorder are sedentary lifestyle and high-fat energy-rich diets. This is a result of fundamental adaptive changes involving the societal and behavioural patterns of modern communities, attributable mainly to increased urbanization and industrialization at the cost of the fading or disappearing traditional ways of living. These traits are themselves significantly influenced by other risk factors, such as BMI, which exhibits great inter-ethnical variability. To begin with, BMI is determined by the distribution of the body fat, which in turn depends on age and sex. The average body fat is known to differ among ethnic populations, as suggested by studies demonstrating that most Asian ethnicities have higher average body fat percentage than whites of the same age and BMI [63–65], for example. These variations appear to be a result of the distribution of body fat for a given BMI. A study in the Singaporean population established differences among its ethnic subpopulations in the association of the CETP variants, Taq1B and -629C>A, with plasma HDL-cholesterol in which the BMI was uniformly linked to disease [59]. The adverse health outcomes associated with these variations are often accompanied by additional complexities, especially since the depth of their relationships can also differ by ethnicity. To add to the intricacy of the problem, the relationship of BMI and such adverse health outcomes involves additional complexities of displaying intra-ethnical variations. For example, among white populations, Europeans have been reported to have a higher percentage of body fat at a given BMI than whites in the USA [63, 66], and a study in the Chinese showed lower average BMI levels among rural compared to urban populations [64, 67]. Thus, the BMI levels may also differ considerably among subpopulations within an ethnic group because of prevailing environmental and lifestyle conditions. Given the variations in the ratios of body fat for a given BMI [64–66], some of these studies have led to the notion that Asians may be predisposed to a greater risk of clinical events, such as acquiring hypertension and cardiovascular disease, despite having lower BMI levels than Caucasians [63, 67–70]. Taken together, these data imply that the global impact of obesity on hyperlipidemia is similar across ethnicity, while that of the BMI may differ considerably even within an ethnic group, since the relationship between BMI and percentage of body fat depends on age and sex, and differs across ethnic groups [63, 65]. Gender has also been implicated, whereby for example, female veterans have been shown to display higher LDL-cholesterol than males [71]. Hence, the penetrance of their influence is ultimately dependent on their distribution by ethnicity. Differences in lipid profiles, prevalence of dyslipidemia and their risk factors can also be explained as product of combined effects of lifestyle and genetic factors [72]. Such inter-ethnical differences in the prevalence of obesity, cholesterol, hypertension and diabetes have similarly been ascribed to socio-economic effects and lifestyle changes [73]. The direct influence of the different risk traits on dyslipidemia can also vary within an ethnic group in presence of racial admixturing. All these variations will affect the appropriateness of managing dyslipidemic disorders in an ethnicity-dependent fashion.

3. Drug therapy of hypercholesterolemia

3.1. Anti-lipidemic agents

Anti-lipidemic agents are entities that are employed to enhance the reduction of circulating lipid levels. These agents can reduce LDL-cholesterol level and/or triglyceride levels, or facilitate the elevation of HDL-cholesterol, thereby preventing both the primary and secondary symptoms of CAD. These agents fall into one of the following categories: (a) bile acid sequestrants, (b) cholesterol absorption inhibitors, (c) 3-hydroxy-3-methylglutaryl coenzyme A (HMG-CoA) reductase inhibitors, (d) fibric acid derivatives, (e) proprotein convertase subtilisin/kexin type 9 (PCSK9) inhibitors and (f) miscellaneous agents (**Table 2**).

3.1.1. Bile acid sequestrants

Bile acid sequestrants are a group of polymeric ion exchange resins that disrupt the enterohepatic circulation of cholesterol-containing bile acids by combining with bile components and preventing their re-absorption from the gut. These drugs are not absorbed following oral administration. They also do not undergo hydrolysis by digestive enzymes or become adsorbed into systemic circulation, but rather bind to bile acids in the intestines and prevent their reabsorption into the body. Hence, they are employed to reduce LDL-cholesterol levels by binding to cholesterol-containing bile acids in the intestines. Since the bound complex is insoluble, it is excreted in faeces. Accordingly, the liver is triggered to produce more bile acids, subsequently reducing the levels of circulating LDL-cholesterol. A decrease in bile leads to an increase in hepatic synthesis of bile acids from cholesterol, and a depletion of cholesterol increases LDLR activity, therefore increasing the removal of LDL-cholesterol from circulation.

Class	Drugs (examples)	Function	Mechanism	Metabolizing pathways/ enzymes
Bile acid sequestrants	Cholestyramine Colesevelam Colestipol	Binding to bile acids in intestines leading to LDLC reduction	Prevent resorption, decrease in bile acid; increase in hepatic synthesis of bile acids	P-glycoprotein; currently no CYP450-related information available
Cholesterol absorption inhibitors	Ezetimibe	Reduce dietary and biliary cholesterol absorption through the intestines	increased hepatic LDLR activity, thereby leading to increase clearance of LDLC	UGT-glucuronidation; Currently no CYP450-related information available
Fibric acid derivatives	Bezafibrate Clofibrate Gemfibrozil Fenofibrate Clinofibrate	Decrease formation of VLDL -cholesterol and triglycerides and an elevation in HDLC	Activating PPARs inducing transcription of gene that facilitate lipid metabolism	Hepatic, CYP3A4; P-glycoprotein; UDP-glucuronosyltransferases
Statins (HMG-CoA reduc tase inhibi tors)	Atorvastatin Fluvastatin Pravastatin Lovastatin Simvastatin Rosuvastatin	Increase in LDL membrane receptors, and therefore clear ance of LDLC from blood	inhibit the function of the HMG CoA enzyme; P-glyco protein substrates	Hepatic; CYP3A4; CYP3A5; CYP2C9; CYP2C19; CYP1A1; CYP2C8; CYP2D6; UGT-glucuronidation
PCSK9 inhibitors	Alirocumab Evolcumab	Antibodies, preven ting LDLR destruction	inhibits PCSK9 Increase LDLR availability	Reticuloendothelial system? Currently no CYP450-related data
Nicotinic acid agents	Niacin Niacor Slo-Niacin	Reduction in LDLC and increase in total HDL; decrease ApoB-100 levels	Precursors for NAD and NADP involved in hydrogen transfer processes	Hepatic; currently no CYP450-related information available
CETP inhibitors	Torcetrapid Anacetrapid Evacetrapid	Blocking all major plasma CETP lipid transfer functions	Induction of non-productive enzyme complex with HDL	Currently no CYP450-related information available

ApoB-100, apolipoprotein B-100; CETP, cholesteryl ester transport protein; CVD, atherosclerotic cardiovascular disease; HEFH, heterozygous familial hypercholesterolemia; HDL, high-density lipoprotein; HDLC, high-density lipoprotein-cholesterol; HMG-CoA; 3-hydroxy-3-methylglutaryl coenzyme A; HOFH, homozygous familial hypercholesterolemia; LDL, low-density lipoprotein; LDLC, low-density lipoprotein cholesterol; LDLR, low-density lipoprotein receptor; NAD, nicotinamide adenine dinucleotide; NADP, NAD phosphate; PCSK9, proprotein convertase subtilin/kinase subtype 9; PPARs; peroxisome proliferator-activated receptors; TG, triglycerides; UGT, uridine 5'diphosphate-glucuronosyltransferase.

Table 2. Summary of the function, functional mechanism and metabolic pathways of anti-lipidemic drugs.

3.1.2. Cholesterol absorption inhibitors

Cholesterol absorption inhibitors, such as ezetimibe, belong to a group of chemicals known as monobactams. They decrease the amount of intestinal cholesterol that is delivered to the liver by reducing the absorption of dietary and biliary cholesterol through the intestines. Thus, these drugs exert their effects by lowering both LDL-cholesterol and total cholesterol. Specifically, ezetimibe selectively inhibits the intestinal absorption of cholesterol and related phytosterols, thereby leading to a decrease in cholesterol clearance from the blood. It does not, however, inhibit cholesterol synthesis in the liver. A reduction in cholesterol levels delivered to the liver results in increased hepatic LDLR activity. This, in turn, enhances the clearance of LDL-cholesterol. The use of ezetimibe is called for especially in individuals who cannot take statins or as additional drug in cases where a need arises to maintain a low statin drug dose because of side effects. Ezetimibe is primarily metabolized via glucuronide conjugation.

3.1.3. Fibric acid derivatives

Fibric acid derivatives are broad-spectrum lipid lowering drugs, whose main action leads not only to a decrease in triglyceride levels, but also a reduction in LDL-cholesterol levels, thereby contributing to the elevation of HDL-cholesterol. The drugs are believed to activate the peroxisome proliferator-activated receptor alpha (PPAR-α). This protein activates the lipoprotein lipase, ultimately resulting in decreased formation of VLDL cholesterol and triglycerides and an elevation in HDL-cholesterol. The three drugs, bezafibrate, clofibrate and gemfibrozil, are hepatically metabolized. Clofibrate is metabolized and rapidly de-esterified in the gastrointestinal tract or through first pass metabolism to its active form clofibrate acid (chlorophenoxy isobutyric acid). Gemfibrozil undergoes UDP-glucuronidation (oxidation) through different isoforms of the UDP-glucuronosyltransferase to gemfibrozil 1-b-glucuronide, to eventually form a hydroxymethyl and a carboxyl metabolite. However, the enzymes responsible for bezafibrate metabolism have not been identified yet. Currently, no metabolic pathway has been defined for fenofibrate and clinofibrate yet.

3.1.4. The 3-hydroxy-3-methylglutaryl coenzyme A reductase inhibitors

The 3-hydroxy-3-methylglutaryl coenzyme A (HMG CoA) reductase (HMGCR) inhibitors, also known as statins, are drugs that reduce cholesterol synthesis in the liver by competitively inhibiting the HMGCR activity. A decrease in cholesterol production leads to an increase in the number of membrane LDLRs, which enhances the clearance of LDL-cholesterol from circulation. This, in turn, leads to an increased hepatic LDLR expression and greater uptake of LDL-cholesterol from plasma, thereby reducing the production of very low-density lipoprotein (VLDL), the precursor of LDL. The net statin dose-dependent reductions in LDL cholesterol are 20–60%, accompanied by some reductions in plasma triglyceride and a small rise in HDL-cholesterol.

The most commonly used statins are simvastatin and artovastatin. Until recently atorvastatin was considered the most effective statin available for decreasing LDL given in daily doses of 10–80 mg. Furthermore, the higher dose was shown to decrease serum triglycerides by 45% in individuals with hypertriglyceridemia. However, rosuvastatin appears to be even more effective than atorvastatin in lowering LDL-cholesterol over its licensed dose range of 10–40 mg, although there appears to be no significant difference between 40 mg rosuvastatin and 80 mg atorvastatin in this respect. The advent of statins into anti-lipidemic therapy was triggered by the discovery and deciphering of the role of the LDLR in FH. They were soon found not only to lower the LDL-cholesterol levels, but also to effect a significant reduction in cardiac events and mortality. They are probably the most effective drugs in lowering LDL-cholesterol available to date. They lower both the LDL-cholesterol and risk for cardiovascular disease in a concentration-dependent fashion.

3.1.5. Proprotein convertase sublitisin/kexin type 9 inhibitors

The proprotein convertase sublitisin/kexin type 9 (PCSK9) inhibitors, alirocumab and evolocumab, are human monoclonal antibodies, which act by inhibiting the PCSK9 function to increase the LDLR availability. They are employed primarily for treating adults with HEFH, HOFH or clinical atherosclerotic cardiovascular disease taking other cholesterol lowering medication, but requiring additional lowering of cholesterol. Inhibition of PCSK9 function holds significant promise as a therapeutic option especially for reducing cardiovascular risk.

3.1.6. Cholesteryl ester transport protein inhibitors

The cholesteryl ester transport protein (CETP) inhibitors apparently function by blocking all of the major lipid transfer functions of plasma CETP through an induction of a non-productive complex between the transfer protein and HDL. By inhibiting the CETP function of transferring HDL-cholesterol to the VLDLs or LDLs, they increase the HDL levels and reduce that of the LDLs.

3.1.7. Nicotinic acid agents

The nicotinic acid agents, such as the nicotinic acid (niacin) itself, are water-soluble vitamin B derivatives, which increase the lipoprotein levels in high doses, lower total cholesterol, LDL-cholesterol and triglyceride levels, while raising HDL-cholesterol level. Niacin is a precursor to nicotinamide adenine dinucleotide (NAD) and nicotinamide adenine dinucleotide phosphate (NADP), which are co-factors to several enzymes. These agents are hepatically metabolized. The mechanism involved in their lipid lowering actions in not fully understood yet. It appears to involve several actions, such as a decrease in esterification of hepatic triglycerides.

3.1.8. Combinations and miscellaneous agents in anti-lipidemic therapy

As described above, some of the anti-lipidemic agents target the lowering of LDL-cholesterol, some aim to reduce triglyceride levels, while others assist in raising HDL-cholesterol. They can prevent both primary and secondary symptoms of CAD. However, some patients who are statin-resistant or intolerant do not respond to or do so very weakly for single drug treatment. Combinations of different anti-lipidemic agents, such as niacin or ezetimibe with statins, can lead to significant reduction in the levels of LDL-cholesterol and triglycerides in blood. Treatment with ezetimibe-bile acid sequestrants and statin-gemfibrozil is also available [74]. Anti-lipidemic agents are also available in combination with anti-hypertensive agents. This is consistent with the concept that taking one tablet of such a combination of agents makes it more conducive and easier for patients to take their medications, which in turn increases compliance. Apart from the above-mentioned classes of drugs, several other agents are also employed to treat patients for lowering of LDL-cholesterol and triglycerides as well as raising HDL-cholesterol.

3.2. Influence of ethnicity on patient response to anti-lipidemic therapy

The response (efficacy) of a drug is a product of both its pharmacodynamic and pharmacokinetic characteristics. However, genetic factors also have a significant, albeit less well documented, impact on how individuals respond to drug therapy. Pharmacodynamics is a discipline that characterizes the biochemical and physiological effects of drugs, the mechanisms of drug action and the relationship between drug concentrations and effect. Pharmacokinetics, on the other hand, relates to the interaction of a drug with the body with respect to absorption, distribution, metabolism and excretion (ADME) properties. Hence (pharmaco)dynamically, the effect of the drug will be influenced by structural changes, particularly to receptor proteins and signalling transduction entities, while (pharmaco)kinetically, these effects will be modulated by modifications in entities, particularly enzymes, involved in the bioavailability or excretion of the drug. Hence, polymorphisms in genes encoding proteins that mediate the effects of the anti-lipidemic drugs, such as receptors, as well as in the cholesterol biosynthetic pathways exert a significant impact on the therapeutic outcome of these drugs in a given population. With respect to hyperlipidemia, in particular, structural changes in the majority of the genes involved in the binding of cholesterol to its vehicles, such as the LDLR or apoA1, for example, would affect the dynamics, while those that are involved in its different ADME phases would influence the kinetics. For example, the ARH individuals appear to be more responsive to lipid lowering drugs. Furthermore, patients with ARH resulting from LDLRAP1 mutations are likely to have more severe cardiovascular involvement than the hypercholesterolemia homozygotes, and will also present with lower LDL-cholesterol and higher HDL-cholesterol levels. It is also generally thought that patients with HOFH do not respond well to lipid lowering therapy with statins because they cannot respond to an increased demand for hepatic cholesterol through the up-regulation of the LDLR activity. Variation in response to anti-lipidemic agents has also been linked to polymorphisms in the *CETP, APOE, HMGCR, CLMN* and *APOC1* genes, whereby, for example, APOE genotypes have been associated with differential response to treatment with fenofibrate [75].

The efficacy of a drug is determined not only by its pharmacodynamic state, but also by its pharmacokinetic (ADME) properties. Accordingly, drug metabolism passes through three phases. These include the modification of the drug through interaction with the CYP450 family of enzymes (phase I) to introduce a reactive or polar group. This is followed by the conjugation of the altered substance to a polar compound in phase II reactions. This is then catalysed by a transferase enzyme, such as glutathione S transferases. In the final stage (phase III), the conjugated product may be further processed prior to recognition by efflux transporters and removed from the cells. Hence, the metabolic rate usually determines the duration and intensity of the pharmacological action of an agent.

The CYP450s constitute a multi-gene family of primarily membrane-associated proteins that are expressed in most organ systems and play important roles in the synthesis and biotransformation of hormones, cholesterol and vitamin D, among others, and are engaged in a large and diverse range of enzymatic activities, including the catalysis of organic substrate oxidation [76–78]. Specifically, they constitute the most important metabolizers for anti-lipidemic agents, particularly the HMGCR inhibitors (statins) [79]. The most important CYP450 phase I enzymes in the metabolism of anti-lipidemic drugs are the CYP2C and CYP3A subfamily as well as the CYP2D6 and CYP1A1 enzymes. **Table 3** gives examples of some of the important CYP variants in anti-lipidemic therapy. These enzymes vary in the extent of their involvement in drug metabolism, whereby some metabolize a limited cohort while others process multiple substrates. Thus, for example, atorvastatin is metabolized through at least two CYP450s, CYP3A4 and CYP3A5, to the ortho- and parahydroxylated metabolites, all of which are capable of inhibiting the HMGCR activity, while fluvastatin is metabolized hepatically via hydroxylation to the 6-hyroxyfluvastatin, 5-hydroxyfluvastatin and N-deisopropylfluvastatin by the CYP2C9, but is also thought to be metabolized to a lesser extent to the 5-hydroxyfluvastatin by a number of other subtypes including the CYP1A1, CYP2C8, CYP2D6 and CYP3A4. It undergoes glucuronidation via the uridine diphosphate glucuronyltransferase (UGT) enzyme system. Pravastatin appears to be hepatically metabolized by CYP2C9, CYP2D6 and CYP3A4 with no notable effect on its overall activity and elimination. Simvastatin is similarly hepatically metabolized to its β-hydroxyacid metabolite through CYP3A4. Rosuvastatin is only slightly metabolized to the rosuvastatin 5 S-lactone by CYP2C9 and N-desmethylrosuvastatin by the CYP2C9 and CYP2C19. Lovastatin is hepatically metabolized primarily to the β-hydroxyacid, through as yet undefined enzymes, and undergoes glycosylation by the P-glycoprotein pathway. In the presence of a genetic change in the metabolizing enzymes, these intended therapeutic end-point may be adversely affected leading to lack of activity or even enhanced side effects of the drugs.

The activity of each enzyme encoded by the combination of CYP450 alleles is categorized as one of five possible phenotypes: normal (NM), poor (PM), intermediate (IM), rapid (RM) and ultra-rapid (URM) metabolizers [80]. Alleles that lead to defective, qualitatively altered, diminished or enhanced rates of drug metabolism have been identified for most of the CYP450s. Defective alleles are usually a product of gene deletions, or conversion, whereby pseudo-gene and single nucleotide polymorphisms cause frameshift, mis-sense, nonsense or splice site mutations. Thereby, homozygous forms lead to a total absence of an active enzyme and impaired ability to metabolize drugs. The PM phenotype is caused by 'loss-of-function' alleles, while URMs are a result of a duplication or amplification of an active gene, and IM are often heterozygous or carry alleles with mutations that decrease enzyme activity only moderately. Star nomenclature is commonly used in describing the various allelic subtypes of the enzyme. Accordingly, the *1 is designated as normal (commonly referred to as wild-type or fully functional) and subsequent variant alleles are numbered in the order that they are identified and characterized. Each pharmacogenetic allele may include several SNPs in form of a haplotype, rather than a single site mutation. Thus, functional changes in the encoding genes lead to enzymes with decreased/increased activity or lack of enzyme expression/activity through various molecular mechanisms. Furthermore, the incidence of a poor or slow metabolizer phenotype for a given enzyme triggered by allelic variants may vary significantly between populations.

Gene	Common name	RS ID	Arabs	Eur	CEU	Jap	Chin	Afr	Asians
CYP1A1	CYP1A1*2C_2454A>G(I462V)	rs1048943	0.061	0.031	0.232	0.209	0.232	0.036	0.256
	CYP1A1*4_2452C>A (T461N)	rs1799814	0.829	0.030	0.025	0.011	0.000	0.003	n.a.
	CYP1A1_134G>A (G45D)	rs4646422	0.001	0.000	0.000	0.168	0.139	0.000	0.14
	CYP1A1_1412T>C (I286T)	rs4987133	0.965	n.a.	0.004	0.000	0.012	0.000	n.a.
CYP1A2	CYP1A2*1C_-3860G>A (Promoter)	rs2069514	0.915	0.020	0.081	ND	ND	0.313	0.242
	CYP1A2*1F_-163C>A (Promoter)	rs762551	0.699	0.320	0.279	0.395	0.337	0.434	0.312
	CYP1A2*1K_-729C>T (Promoter)	rs12720461	0.958	n.a.	0.000	0.000	0.023	0.000	0.023
	CYP1A2*1K_-739T>G (Promoter)	rs2069526	0.096	n.a.	0.004	0.041	0.09	0.128	0.093
CYP2C8	CYP2C8*2	rs11572103	n.a.	0.004	0.000	0.000	0.000	0.190	n.a..
	CYP2C8*3	rs1050968, rs11572080	n.a.	0.118	0.137	0.000	0.000	0.000	0.000
	CYP2C8*4 (C>G)	rs1058930	n.a.	0.058	0.066	0.000	0.000	0.004	0.000
	CYP2C8*8	rs72558195	n.a.	0.001	n.a.	n.a.	n.a.	n.a.	n.a.
CYP2C9	CYP2C9*11_42542C>T (R335W)	rs28371685	0.996	0.002	0.022	0.006	ND	0.024	0.000
	CYP2C9*2_3608C>T (R144C)	rs1799853	0.852	0.124	0.104	0.000	0.000	0.008	n.a.
	CYP2C9*3_42614A>C (I359L)	rs1057910	0.944	0.059	0.058	0.023	0.047	0.000	0.044
	CYP2C9*6 (−/A)	rs9332131	N.A.	0.000	0.000	N.A.	N.A.	0.008	N.A.
CYP2C18	CYP2C18_c. *31C>T (3′UTR)	rs2860840	0.269	0.384	0.384	0.224	0.233	0.004	0.233
	CYP2C18_c. *592C>A (3′UTR)	rs1326830	0.009	0.042	0.000	0.215	0.174	0.021	n.a.
	CYP2C18_c.204T>A (Y68X)	rs41291550	0.012	n.a.	0.006	0.106	0.037	0.064	n.a.
CYP2C19	CYP2C19*17_-806C>T	rs12248560	0.744	0.224	0.217	0.000	0.022	0.275	0.022
	CYP2C19*2	rs4244285	n.a.	0.145	0.155	0.284	0.256	0.144	n.a.
	CYP2C19*3	rs4986893, rs57081121	n.a.	0.000	n.a.	n.a.	n.a.	0.002	0.058
CYP2D6	CYP2D6*4	rs3892097	n.a.	0.186	n.a.	n.a.	n.a.	0.061	0.006
	CYP2D6*17	rs28371706(T); rs16947 (A)	n.a.	0.002	n.a.	n.a.	n.a.	0.218	0.000
SCLO1B1	SLCO1B1*5	rs4149056	n.a.	0.161	0.158	0.110	0.151	0.014	0.128
UGT1A1	UGT1A1*28	rs4148323, rs8175347	n.a.	0.007	0.000	0.111	0.200	0.001	0.161

Minor allele distribution of CAD-related variation among different ethnic groups. Asians, represents studies done in other (non-Japanese, non-Chinese) ethnicities; Afr, Africans, predominantly Yoruba; Arabs, ethnic Middle East Arabs; Chin, Chinese, primarily the Han population; CEU, Caucasians; EUR, Europeans; Jap, Japanese; RS ID, DBSNP ID.

Table 3. Ethnicity and anti-hypercholesterolemia therapy–related gene variants.

The CYP2Cs involved in anti-lipidemic drug metabolism consist of four isoform members, CYP2C8, CYP2C9, CYP2C18 and CYP2C19, which are also thought to metabolize approximately 20% of all clinically used drugs [81]. The CYP2C8 gene resides within a cluster of CYP450 genes on chromosome 10q23.33. In liver microsomes, it is involved in an NADPH-dependent electron transport pathway engaged in the oxidation of structurally unrelated compounds. It exhibits at least 16 allelic forms denoted *1A, *1B, *1C and *2-*14 (http://www.cypalleles.ki.se/). At least five of these (*2, *3, *4, *8 and *14) encode proteins with decreased enzyme activity. The distribution of variant alleles of *CYP2C8* gene differs among ethnic populations [4]. The *CYP2C8*2*, the variant most common in Africans, is related to a poor metabolizer phenotype (PM) in subjects carrying at least one copy of the defective allele [4, 9]. Poor metabolizers experience a longer drug half-life [12] and increased adverse side effects.

The CYP2C9, which constitutes the main enzyme for rate-limiting metabolism of fluvastatin, pravastatin and rosuvastatin, appears to have the largest impact on the dose requirements, and is thought to hydroxylate about 16% of therapeutically used drugs. The gene resides on chromosome 10q23.33. It exists in at least 66 allelic forms (*1A-D, *2A-C, *3A, B, *4-*60) (http://www.cypalleles.ki.se/), whereby the vast majority encode proteins with decreased activity. Hence, the impact of its variants on anti-lipidemic drug therapy is of significant consequence. Of special interest are those with a narrow therapeutic index, where impairment in CYP2C9 metabolic activity might cause difficulties in dose adjustment as well as toxicity [82]. *In vitro* data have demonstrated an association of the *CYP2C9*2* and *3 alleles with significant reduction in intrinsic clearance of a variety of CYP2C9 substrates compared with the wild-type CYP2C9*1. However, the extent of these reductions appears to be highly substrate-dependent [83]. In addition, multiple *in vivo* investigations and clinical case reports have associated genotypes expressing the *CYP2C9*2* and *3 alleles with significant reductions in both the metabolism and daily dose requirements of selected CYP2C9 substrates [83]. For example, an allelic variant causing a Leu359 to Ile359 substitution has been implicated in the decreased metabolic clearance of various therapeutic agents [81, 83]. Similarly, the variants coding for R144C (*2) and I359L (*3) amino acid substitutions have been suggested to exert significant functional effects and exhibit appreciably high population frequencies. Accordingly, individuals expressing these variant genotypes also appear to be significantly more susceptible to adverse events with the narrow therapeutic index agents, especially during the initiation of therapy [84]. The pharmacokinetics of fluvastatin enantiomers were found to depend on the CYP2C9 genotypes [85], leading to the proposition for potential clinical utilization of the later in adjustment of drug dose of the former [85].

Probably the most familiar of the CYP2C subfamilies with respect to their impact on drug efficacy is the CYP2C19 [86, 87]. The encoding *CYP2C19* gene is located on chromosome 10q23.33. At least 49 allelic forms (*1A-C, 2A-H, *2J, *3A-C, *4A, B, *5A, B *6-*35) have been reported for this gene. The important phenotypes for its anti-lipidemic therapy include the ultra-rapid (URM; *17), extensive (EM), intermediate (IM) and poor (*2 or *3) metabolizers as well as loss-of-function (*4). Its PM phenotype is important in statin therapy, whereby these individuals quite frequently experience exaggerated drug response and side effects at standard doses.

The CYP2D6 (debrisoquine/sparteine hydroxylase) acts on about 25% of all prescription medications, including the drugs that are employed in management of dyslipidemic disorders. The encoding *CYP2D6* gene itself, located on chr22q13.2, is highly polymorphic, and several mutations leading to the absence of a functional enzyme have been identified [80]. Currently, there are more than 77 alleles (including *1A-E, *1XN, *2A-H, *2J-M, *2XN, *3A, B, *4A-H, *4J-P, *5, *6A-D, *7-9, *9X2, *10A-D, *10X2K, *11-13, *14A, B, *15-17, *17XN, *18-35) described for this locus. Although the gene appears in several polymorphic forms, probably only the six most common defective alleles will predict its phenotype with almost absolute certainty [88]. The PMs include *2 - *6, *10, *17, *29 *35 and *41, whereby the null alleles do not encode a functional protein with detectable residual enzyme activity. Combinations of altered alleles have been described resulting from substitutions, deletions or copy number changes, such as duplications of the entire gene leading to variant metabolizer phenotypes ranging from PM to URM. The CYP2D6 PM phenotypes are important for patients taking anti-lipidemic agents, as they may exhibit poor tolerance to these drugs [89]. Like the CYP2C19, PMs of drugs metabolized through the CYP2D6 often experience exaggerated drug response and side effects at standard statin doses. Clinical consequences of the CYP2D6 polymorphism may manifest either in form of adverse drug reactions or altered drug response. It has been demonstrated, for example, that the pharmacokinetics of fluvastatin enantiomers depend on the CYP2C9 genotypes, leading to potentially toxic bioactivation reactions [85].

The *CYP3A4* and *CYP3A5* form part of a CYP450 gene cluster constituting a group of heme-thiole mono-oxygenases on chr7q21.1. The CYP3A4 protein localizes to the endoplasmic reticulum and its expression is induced by glucocorticoids and some pharmacological agents. The enzyme is apparently involved in the metabolism of about 50% of the drugs in use today, including several HMGCR inhibitors, through the hydroxylation process. This process is often followed by dehydrogenation leading to more complex metabolites [90]. However, most of the drugs undergo deactivation by CYP3A4 either directly or by facilitated excretion from the body. Alternative splicing of the gene results in many transcript variants. Thus far, about 45 alleles (*1A-H, *1J-T, *2-14, *15A-B, *17, *18A-B *19-26) have been described, majority of which result in decreased function of the enzyme. The other member, CYP3A5, is localized to the endoplasmic reticulum in liver tissue. In liver microsomes, the CYP3A5 is involved in NADPH-dependent electron transport pathways. At least two pseudo-genes of the CYP3A5 gene have been identified at this locus. It exists in about 25 allelic forms (*1A-E, *2, *3A-L, *4-*10), the majority of which encode proteins with severely attenuated enzyme activity. Furthermore, the CYP1A1 resides on chromosome 15q24.1. To date, 16 alleles, *1, *2A-C, 3-*13, have been described, but their characteristics have not been fully elucidated yet.

Several protein families, other than the CYPs, such as the uridine 5'diphosphate-glucuronosyltransferase (UGTs) and solute carrier organic anion transporters (OATPs, SLCs), also contribute to the ADME processes of anti-lipidemic agents. The UGT family is responsible for catalysing the glucuronidation and transfer of a wide range of drugs including statins, environmental chemicals and endogenous substances. The major UGTs include the UGT1A1, UGT2B7 and UGT2B15. Several non-functional alleles have been described for the UGT1A1 including UGT1A1*6, UGT1A1*60 and UGT1A1*93. However, polymorphisms of this gene have been primarily associated with disease manifestation, rather than drug response. The SLCs are key determinants of ADME of various drugs, including statins, as a result of their broad substrate specificity and tissue distribution. Several alleles have also been described, which form haplotypes leading to altered transport activity. Thereby, the SLCO1A2 mediates the sodium-independent transport of organic anions and conjugated and unconjugated bile acids.

3.3. Impact of ethnicity on the role of genetic variations in anti-lipidemic drug metabolizing enzymes

Apart from changes in the metabolic enzymes themselves, variations also exist in the impact of these changes on anti-lipidemic therapy among different ethnicities [91–97]. These variations can be manifested in various ways, including changes in drug potency or metabolism and the pharmacokinetics of the drug may in turn be attributable to alterations in polymorphic traits of metabolic pathways. The impact of ethnicity becomes particularly apparent in the way individuals respond to drug therapy of dyslipidemia, in which multiple researchers have demonstrated great variability in the distribution of these genetic variants by ethnicity. For example, in a number of studies in the USA, differences have been described in variants both among indigenous populations as well as in comparison with African, Asian and European populations. Such differences were documented, for example, between Oriental, Caucasians, Saudis and American black populations, in the prevalence of defective CYP2C19 alleles [98]. Thereby, PMs represented approximately 3–5% of Caucasians and African-Americans, but 12–100% of Asian groups [81]. Similar variations have also been reported among Caucasians, Africans and East Asians [99], whereby higher CYP2C19*2 and *3 (PMs) were observed in Mexicans than in African-Americans, whites, East Asians and Southeast Asians [100], among the Chinese ethnic populations [101–103], between Sri Lankan and European populations [104], between Hungarian and Roman populations [105] in a US pan-ethnic groups of whites, African American, Hispanics and Ashekenazi Jewish populations [106] as well as Pacific individuals and New Zealand Europeans [103], among others. The CYP2C19*2 also appears to be more common in Finland and Spain, respectively, than in the UK, while Asians appear to exhibit low CYP2C19*2 and CYP2C19*12, but higher CYP2C19*2 frequencies compared to the UK residents of European ethnicity [107]. Both variants have been found to be also more frequent in East Asians and even higher in native populations from Oceania compared to Mediterranean, South European and Middle Eastern ethnicities. The observation of an increase in the Oceanians has been explained by genetic drift in the Pacific Islands [108]. Similar differences have also been reported between the Malaysian Chinese and Caucasians and in Israeli individuals of different ethnic backgrounds [109, 110]. Like the *2 and *3, significant ethnic difference have also been observed in the frequency of the *17 (UM) variant that leads to very rapid metabolism of its substrates among various groups in a pan-ethnic study including Mediterranean, South European and Middle Eastern than in East Asians [108]. Furthermore, although the role of CYP2C18 in drug metabolism remains obscure, it was recently suggested that defective *CYP2C19*3* and *CYP2C18*1* alleles are completely linked, implying that a *CYP2C19*3* PM is a CYP2C18 PM and vice versa [111]. A gender-dependent activity of the CYP2C19 and higher incidence of PMs was also described in Koreans as compared to Swedish [112].

The gene encoding the *CYP2C9* also harbours numerous variations which have increasingly been acknowledged as determinants of the metabolic phenotype underlying inter-individual and inter-ethnic differences in response to drug therapy [91, 92]. Existing data suggests that the CYP2C9*2 and *3 alleles are present in approximately 35% of Caucasian individuals, but significantly less so in African-American and Asian populations [83]. Similar differences have been observed between Amerindians and Admixed or European populations [113] as well as Swedes and Koreans [114]. Thus, for example, *CYP2C9**2 and *3 variants were more frequent among white populations than in Africans and Asians, while *CYP2C9**2 was detected only in Asians [115]. The CYP2C9*2 frequency also appears to be lower in South Asians compared to the UK residents of European ethnicity [107], but more common in Finland and Spain than in the UK [107], comparatively lower among Mexican-Americans compared to Spaniards [116]. Its distribution also varies between Beninese and Belgian populations [117], Ethiopians and Italian Caucasians [118], Amerindians and European admixtures [119], Iranians, African and Eastern Asian populations [120], Hungarian and Roma populations [121], as well as among the Chinese minority ethnicities [101], ethnic Jewish groups [122] and Mexican ethnicities [123, 124]. Interestingly, to date, the *CYP2C9*4* appears to have been exclusively identified in Japanese patients, while the *CYP2C9*5* and *6 were only found with a low allelic frequency among African-Americans, respectively [115].

Another genetically polymorphic CYP2C of potential clinical relevance with respect to anti-lipidemia therapy is the *CYP2C8*. Differences in the prevalence of the CYP2C8*2 allele have been described between the Bantu and San populations in Botswana [125], between Caucasian Europeans and South Asians [126], among the Chinese minority populations [127], South Indian populations, African, European Chinese and Japanese [128], Ghanaian, Caucasians and Asians [129], as well as among African-American, European-Americans, Japanese, Han Chinese and Koreans [130]. Interestingly, Caucasian Americans also display large variability in CYP2C8 and CYP2C9 suspected to be along ethnic ancestry, and a higher frequency is thought to exist among Caucasian Americans with South European ancestry than with North European ancestry. Notably, differences in the prevalence of CYP2C8*3, CYP2C9*2 and CYP2C9*3 alleles have also been reported between Chinese and Japanese individuals, East and South Asians as well as among Caucasian Europeans [126]. Furthermore, apart from inter-ethnical differences, there appears to be also intra-ethnic variability in the CYP2C8 and CYP2C9 allele frequencies [126]. This implies therefore that, for example, Asians or Caucasians cannot be conceived as homogeneous populations with respect to these enzyme families.

The CYP2D6 can convert statins to a metabolizer that has a greater effect. It also exhibits multiple non-functional variants. In contrast to CYP2C19 distribution, CYP2D6 PMs are reportedly more frequent among Europeans than in Asians, while differences were also observed between Chinese and Caucasians in CYP2D6 PMs and IMs [109]. It has been suggested that about 10% of Caucasians lack any CYP2D6 activity due to deletions and frameshift or splice site mutations in the gene. The CYP2D6*4 appears to be the most common PM among Europeans and to be more frequent in the UK than in Spain and Finland [107]. Furthermore, approximately 3% of Middle-Europeans and 29% of Ethiopians display gene duplication, leading to elevated URM phenotype. Distribution of CYP2D6 PM has also been reported to differ between the Russian, Yemente and Israeli Arab ethnic groups [131], Tibetian and Han populations [132], the Amerindians and Asians in Venezuela [133] and among some Chinese ethnic minorities [101, 103, 134]. In Mexico, differences have been observed in CYP2D6*4 between Caucasians and Mexican Americans [135], while in Israel such variation in CYP2D6*4, *10 and *17 alleles and CYP2D6 duplications have been described between the Ethiopian, Sephardic Beduoin and Yemente Jews [136]. Prevalence of CYP2D6 UM in the Mediterranean population was higher than those from North Europe [137], in the Mestizo than in Amerindian and Afro-Caribbean population in a Costa Rican study [138] and in the Mediterranean compared to Northern Europe in an Italian study [139]. Similarly, differences exist in the prevalence of defective alleles between Africans and South-East Asians [140] and Hispanics, North American Caucasians and African Americans [141] and between African Americans and Caucasians [142].

The other enzyme sub-families engaged in anti-lipidemic therapy exhibiting significant inter-ethnical variation in defective alleles are the CYP3A4/5 gene cluster [143, 144]. The CYP3A4*19 appears to be frequent in Hispanics, while differences have been described in CYP3A4*18 among the different ethnic Chinese minorities [101, 145]. Also variations have been observed in CYP3A4*IB and CYP3A5*3 between Brazilians of African and European descents [146, 147], between African-Americans and Caucasians [148, 149] and between Indian, Malay, Chinese and Caucasians in Singapore [150, 151]. In contrast, in Indo-Pakistanis, for example, it has been reported that, with the exception of the CYP3A4*1B, the proportion of patients without a CYP3A4 polymorphism appears low.

The CYP1A constitutes a gene family that has been implicated in both drug metabolism and disease. Thus, the gene contains at least four major polymorphisms that exhibit population distribution that is dependent on ethnicity. Among the Chinese, variations have been observed in the CYP1A2 distribution among a number of ethnicities [152]. In European studies, Hungarians showed elevated rapid metabolizing tendencies compared with the Romans [153]. The CYP1F2*1F was found to be more frequent in Mexican Amerindians than Mestizos in a Mexican study [154], while differences in frequency were also reported among ethnic groups in Singapore [155], between Taiwanese, Caucasians and African Americans [156], while Ethiopians appeared to display at least twice the variations found in all other populations combined. A significant association between CYP1A*2c and triglyceride level has been described in Mexican Amerindian Tarahumaras compared to the Tepehuanos [157, 158]. It has also been suggested that CYP1A1*3 may be specific for individuals of African descent, while the CYP1A1*2 is closely linked to Asian ethnicity but less so to Caucasian [159].

Inter-ethnical variation in the distribution of genetic alleles is not limited to the CYP450s only, but is rather a general phenomenon for the majority of proteins involved in the bio-distribution, transport, metabolism and excretion of all drugs and pharmaceutical agents. One of such protein families important for anti-lipidemic drugs is the UGT. Polymorphisms of this gene have been primarily associated with disease manifestation, and only scanty ethnicity-based studies are currently available. One such study in the Chinese has shown heterogeneity among different ethnic groups [160]. Furthermore, differences have also been reported in the prevalence of the UGT1A1*28 between Caucasians and Asians [161]. Besides, some sex-dependent differences have also been discussed with regard to UGT functionality. They are also believed to be involved in drug-drug interactions. Several cell membrane transporters, such as the anion transport polypeptide (OATP) 1B1, encoded by the SLCO1B1 gene, can influence the disposition of statins. They are key determinants of ADME of various drugs as a result of their broad substrate specificity and tissue distribution.

3.3.1. Gene polymorphism, ethnicity and adverse anti-lipidemic drug response

Many of the anti-lipidemic agents frequently exhibit very serious side effects, often leading to discontinuation of the therapeutic regimen. For example, it is thought that statin discontinuation rate due to side effects ranges between 1% and 5%. This is, in the majority of cases, due to the sharing of metabolic pathways by other concomitantly employed drugs, but may also be caused by mutations in the metabolic genes. Adverse effects of anti-lipidemic drugs also include drug resistance and intolerance, which have been linked to genetic polymorphisms in several genes including LDLR, HMGCR, PCSK9, CETP, APOE, P-glycoprotein and OATP, just to name a few. Furthermore, drug dosage requirements are often dependent on ethnic differences as explained, at least in part, by genetic and dietary factors. Such adverse effect would be exacerbated in the presence of defective metabolizing alleles. Several factors, including modes of action, biotransformation routes or concomitant food ingestion, may contribute to these phenomena. Of particular importance in this regard are the CYP450s, which are thought to mediate the majority of unwanted drug effects, as drugs interact with members of this protein family in many different ways, whereby a drug may be metabolized by one or multiple of these enzymes. Thereby, drugs that cause CYP450 metabolic interactions are referred to as either inhibitors or inducers. Such drugs block the metabolic activity of one or more enzymes, whereby the extent of its influence will depend on factors such as dose and the capability of the drug to bind to the enzyme. On the other hand, a drug may induce its metabolizing enzyme. Such enzyme inducers increase the CYP450 activity by increasing its synthesis, often dependent on the half-life of the drug. These factors render the therapy with drugs undergoing metabolism through the CYP450 system complex. Notably, a drug may inhibit the function of an enzyme that metabolizes it, with each cytochrome isozyme responding differently to exogenous chemicals in terms of its induction and inhibition. Typically, individuals with an aberrant CYP450 gene may experience diminished efficacy or increased toxicity in response to particular drugs as a result of the difference in activity levels associated with the variant genotypes. One example is myositis, the most important adverse effect of statins, which may be greatly influenced by the presence of the defective enzymes, such as the CYP2C9, CYP2C19 and CYP3A4 variants. Inhibition of these enzymes often adversely affects the function of the HMGCR inhibitors in different fashions. For example, the CYP3A inhibitors significantly enhance simvastatin plasma concentrations and its active forms. It has also been shown that peak serum levels of simvastatin, which is metabolized solely by CYP3A4, can increase by many times in PMs or with the addition of a potent inhibitor, leading to an increase in the risk of myopathy and rhabdomyolysis at usual doses. The effect of CYP3A4*22 allele is thought to lead to reduced enzyme expression. Combination of non-functional CYP3A5*3 and putative, functionally reduced CYP3A4*1G alleles may predict diminished clearance of CYP3A4 substrates [162]. Carriers of one or more CYP2C variant alleles may be at risk for adverse drug reactions when prescribed together with drugs extensively metabolized by CYP2C9 [115]. Atorvastatin-related rhabdomyolysis and acute renal failure has also been linked OATP1B1 polymorphism and CYP2C19 PMs [163].

The other important enzyme family in anti-lipidemic drug metabolism is the UGT, which may invariably influence drug metabolism through the CYP450 pathways, as demonstrated by the observations that, for example, gemfibrozil exhibits glucuronidation- and reduction-dependent activation to metabolites that inhibit CYP2C8, whereas ezetimibe shows glucuronidation-dependent protection against metabolism-dependent inhibition of CYP3A4. Its polymorphism has also been linked to artovastatin adverse effects by increasing its lactonization in the liver through UGT1A3*2 [164, 165]. While artovastatin lactone is pharmacologically inactive, it is suspected to be a muscle toxic and to cause statin-induced myopathy. Furthermore, UGT1A1*28 has been associated with decreased exposure of artovastatin lactone [166], and also linked to changes in the pharmacokinetics of ezetimibe [167].

Other important gene variants influencing the actions of anti-lipidemic drugs include the CETP-Taq1B and adenosine triphosphate binding cassette transport A1 (ABCA1)-R219K gene polymorphism, which seem to modify the response to lipid lowering therapy with simvastatin or atorvastatin treatment [168, 169]. The frequency of the variant alleles for these drug metabolizing enzymes often differ among ethnic populations. For example, inter-individual variability in statin exposure has been associated with changes in the uptake and efflux of transporter genes. Hence, for each individual, it is important to establish the impact on drug ADME characteristics in order to achieve maximal therapeutic outcomes. Mutations in the solute carrier organic anion transport 1B1 (SCLO1B1) are also known to increase plasma concentrations of simvastatin (and simvastatin-induced myopathy) as well as moderately increase those of pravastatin. In some studies, artovastatin concentrations have been associated with changes in the SCO1B1 [170], although some other investigators failed to report similar effects [171]. SLCO1B1 polymorphism, particularly the SNP rs4149056 (c.521T>C), has also been linked to statin-induced myopathy, while the SLCO1B1*5 allele and female sex have been associated with mild statin-induced side effects [172]. Other anti-lipidemic drugs influenced by the OATP1B1 include ezetimibe [173].

Besides, genes such the *CETP* and multi-drug resistant protein 1 appear to harbour variants that may either enhance LDL-cholesterol or decrease triglyceride and HDL-response to pravastatin treatment [174], while certain *LDLR* and *APOB* mutations and haplotypes reportedly influence the lipid lowering effect of atorvastatin on LDL-cholesterol and apoB levels [175]. Treatment with pravastatin may lead to reduction of cholesterol in individuals harbouring heterozygous variants of the *HMGCR* [176]. These variants have also been implicated in the variations in response to therapy with different anti-lipidemic drugs. An example is that of the *APOE* genotypes associated with response to treatment with fenofibrate [75]. Many drugs are known to inhibit AOTP1B1 function, *in vitro* at least, possibly resulting in, for example, an increase in plasma concentrations of statins. Gemfibrozil has also been shown to increase concentrations of several OATP1B1 substrates.

The sterol regulatory binding proteins 1 and 2 (SREBPs) are transcription factors that regulate lipid metabolism. A recent report also showed that the SREBP-1c polymorphism (G952G) is associated with elevated cholesterol synthesis, and increased response to the effects of ezetimibe on cholesterol absorption [177]. It is thought that inhibition of mevalonate synthesis by statins reduces not only the biosynthesis of cholesterol, but also the production of ubiquinone (CoQ10), which is synthesized in all cells. Reduction of CoQ10 levels causes statin-induced myotoxicity.

3.4. Confounders for the role of ethnicity in hyperlipidemia drug therapy

Since alterations in the metabolizing proteins will affect the pharmacokinetics of a drug, it is also understandable that such changes are likely to play a major role in drug adverse effects. In particular, the effects of anti-lipidemic drugs are influenced in many different directions in the presence of variations in their metabolizing enzymes, which may in turn be also influenced by both modifiable and non-modifiable confounders, including gender and age, as well as concomitant therapies with different families of drugs. For example, one proposed mechanism responsible for a differential effect of statins could be sex-dependent drug clearance, given that the clearance of lipid-soluble statins involves CYP450s and the protein expression can vary by sex. In some animal studies, the metabolic rate of simvastatin was found to be considerably higher in males than in females. The statins might therefore be expected to have a greater clinical effect on males. In contrast, human volunteers showed a lower degree of metabolism of simvastatin and lovastatin in men than in women. Moreover, several epidemiological studies have reported greater reductions in both LDL and total cholesterol in response to statins in women than in men, which presumably could lead to between-sex differences in clearance rates, bioavailability and, consequently, the clinical effects achieved with the same dose of the drug. One study has, for example, indicated that the variability in CYP1A2 activity could be explained by the diet, lifestyle and genetic factors [178]. Some studies even suggest that statin therapy leads to a greater reduction in the risk of cardiovascular events in men than in women with cardiovascular disease. Several of the CYP450s are also implicated in diseases, which may influence the therapeutic outcome with drugs that are metabolized through these enzymes. Besides, diseases such as HIV/AIDS are also known to trigger lipid disorders and need to be considered seriously in their management. It has been shown, for example, that a combination of anti-retroviral therapy is likely to trigger the incidence of metabolic risk factors such as insulin resistance, dyslipidemia, lipoatrophy and abnormal fat distribution. As such, HIV-dyslipidemia is regarded as a common problem linked to an increase in the incidence of cardiovascular disease.

Other confounders include awareness, availability of resources and adequate health service products. Such disparities contribute to inequality in health product supply of any societal community, and to the way management of disease may be accomplished within a society. Some disparities by ethnicity have also been established in the use of pharmacotherapy for hyperlipidemia, orders by physicians, counselling of individual on food intake and exercise [179]. Besides, drug responses are influenced by clinical variables such as age, gender, body weight, general medical condition and liver function. All these factors contribute negatively to attaining national therapeutic goals.

3.5. Ethnicity-gene interactions and future management of hypercholesterolemia

The preceding paragraphs have summarized the causative genes for hyperlipidemia, the diversity in gene variants encoding metabolizing proteins and their distributions in different populations by ethnicity. The summarized data demonstrates that the interactions of these variables do not only influence the expected drug actions, but, more importantly so, also the untoward effects of the therapeutic agents for hypercholesterolemia. It is also evident that, in addition to the complexity of the ethnicity-gene environment interactions, intra-ethnic population admixtures of many modern societies may introduce an element of uncertainty with regards to the interpretation of observations in such population structures. As a result, this may lead to spurious genotype-phenotype associations, which presents a challenge in thriving to unequivocally isolate the ethnic-specific disease-related alleles from those pertaining to multiple population groups. However, the importance of ethnicity in complex disease manifestation such as hyperlipidemia and its pharmacogenetics is now generally acknowledged and cannot be ignored. Rather, it should constitute a central focus of research as a basis for establishing therapeutic goals for targeted disease management. To begin with, existing data reveals that, for example, the disease-causing gene variants and ADME-related alleles are not uniformly distributed among Caucasian, European or individuals from East Asia or Africa. This asymmetric distribution of genotypes implies that we need to decipher their prevalence by ethnicity for us to determine their relevance for any given ethnic group. Hence, knowledge of the extent to which a particular variant may be present within an ethnic population is therefore mandatory in order to establish the chances of success for a personalized therapeutic regimen for anti-hyperlipidemia therapy. The implication for this variability is also that therapeutic modalities have to be predetermined for each individual ethnic population for optimal disease management in any given society. In this regard, the WHO has recommended establishing health action points that may be specific for each nation. On the other hand, there might be some geographic similarities in the prevalence of some variants as shown by some Asian populations sharing unique traits compared to Caucasians, for example. Therefore, it also appears that the distribution of some of these genotypes is heavily influenced by geographic origin. This scenario implies that, while the individuals belonging to these different populations cannot be treated as homogeneous groups, they may nonetheless inherently share some genetic traits that are regulated by geographic demarcations. Hence, the identification and discerning of ethnic-specific variants from such common regional traits should enhance our understanding of the human diversities in genetic traits, and can therefore be exploited more appropriately for therapeutic purposes in the future.

Importantly, the gene-ethnicity relationships are also commonly influenced by confounders, such as age and gender. These two variables are, however, not ethnic-specific, and would independently exert a similar impact on disease or therapy across ethnic groups. On the other hand, however, modifiable traits such as obesity or BMI would be identifiable ethnic-specific traits. Therefore, combinations of these various confounders will impact the relationship of the genotype, ethnicity and disease or therapy in different fashions that cannot be easily transposed from one ethnicity to another. Accordingly, consideration of specific underlying environmental factors is a prerequisite in the management of complex disorders such hyperlipidemia for any given population. With regard to hyperlipidemia specifically, the issue is not made easier by the fact that drugs, such as statins, are invariably metabolized through several CYP450s, and vice versa. Thus, the rate of defects in ADME genes may occupy a unique position in mediating these interactions. Therefore, specific knowledge of the metabolic pathway of these ADME enzyme variants is also key to establishing the success of individual therapy in any ethnic group within societies. Furthermore, understanding of the causal relationship of these polygenic influences on drug dose requirements is vital in reducing inter-patient variability and optimizing anti-lipidemic therapy. Detecting such genetic variations in drug metabolizing enzymes is also particularly important for identifying individuals who may experience adverse drug reactions or lack of drug response. In turn, it should help in the prediction of more individualized loading and maintenance doses for safer drug therapy. In fact, the different isoforms of the ADME enzymes probably present greater challenges with respect to their possible adverse effects and the safety issues than the activity level, not only due to intra-individual, but more so inter-ethnical differences in their prevalence across societies. Ethnic diversity in some of these variants and complex interplay among them will therefore dictate the success of anti-lipidemic therapy in any given population. Thus, for example, dosing for poor metabolizers may have to be significantly modified to meet the ethnic-specific requirements for adequate therapy, which may not necessarily be the case in some societies. On the same note, ethnic-based genetic tests can be used to screen for individuals with poor metabolizer phenotypes, for example, with the ultimate goal of predicting the clinical effects of drugs. Furthermore, apart from drug efficacy, inter-ethnical variations in the prevalence of metabolic genes will naturally also influence drug toxicity. In addition to ethnic-delineable variants, common multi-ethnic variants in important drug metabolizing genes have also been described across ethnicities. This is exacerbated by the fact that some ethnic populations also display a wide range of variations in the frequencies of these polymorphisms, possibly due to population migrations. Put together, the overall clinical merits of a genotype-adapted anti-lipidemic treatment regimen in a patient population can best benefit only if the actual prevalent variants are known for that particular ethnic population. Thus, identification of such ethnic-specific allele frequencies and their phenotypic designation will provide the basis for better clinical management.

Apart from traits directly related to societal structure, gene polymorphism and the reigning classical modifiable risk traits, there are many other events that will determine the outcome of therapeutic management hyperlipidemia. These features include public awareness as well as availability of and access to information or national resources. To begin with, it has been shown that the difference in the availability of health insurance may influence the way patients of different ethnic groups respond to treatment. Furthermore, in many communities there is a suffocating lack of data on the prevalence of the important disease-causing or therapy-related genotypes. Unfortunately, thus far, the phenotypic expression has been studied primarily in Caucasians and a few other ethnicities, but only poorly so in developing or semi-developed countries, such as Africa of the Arab world. Yet by virtue of consanguinity and inbreeding in some of these societies, for example, the distribution pattern of clinically important variants may differ considerably in such communities compared to others, as a result of disparity in Hardy-Weinberg distribution principal. Hence, there is acute need to characterize the prevalence of such variants in such ethnic populations, as they will almost certainly always be unique in a particular society. For dyslipidemia specifically, this complexity is compounded by the lack of community awareness reining in developing countries. Besides, often there are many inconsistences in the data pertaining to different ethnic groups within the same geographical regions. This naturally leads to disparity in the effectiveness of therapy in such societies. One study suggested, for example, that the disparities in the use of pharmacotherapy for hyperlipidemia, physician-ordered or provided cholesterol screening, diet and exercise counselling by specialists may be partly a result of lack of information [179]. Awareness influences compliance, and compliance is a key determinant of successful drug therapy. Furthermore, compliance to drug therapy is influenced by a number of other factors, including volume of drugs to be consumed and rate of daily drug intake, and possibly even gender. Recently, a gender difference in lipid control due to non-adherence has been described [180]. Moreover, apart from the cited studies pointing to differences among ethnic groups, there is also a large amount of data failing to replicate the reports of such genotype-related effects in the same ethnic populations. This may be attributable to several factors, including admixture and lack of information. These will in turn contribute to intra-ethnical variations in the management of drug treatment in a given community.

Availability or lack of resources and adequate health service products also play a central role in the outcome of dyslipidemia therapy. For example, it has been shown that the difference in the availability of health insurance may influence the way patients of different ethnic groups may respond to treatment. In the USA, for example, variations across states in health insurance and racial/ethnicity mixture have been associated with variations in the management of hyperlipidemia. Thus, less-insured states may be less effective, whereas those with more private, Medicare or Medicaid coverage may be more effective. In states with proportionately more African-Americans versus Hispanics, lipid medications have also been found to be prescribed differently [181]. Such disparities contribute to inequality in health product supply of any societal community and therefore to the way management of dyslipidemic disorders may be accomplished within that society. Indeed, such environmental factors will have an impact on disease management that often goes unnoticed. Other environmental factors include access to education, information or resources within the different ethnic populations, whose importance can hardly be overstated. For example, in the USA the native Hawaiians are regarded as the least educated proportionally and the lowest portion of the ladder of socio-economic strata relative to most ethnic groups in the USA, which may explain some of the remarkable differences compared to other groups. One problem is the issue of availability of basic information on disease risk factors and involvement in decision making for therapy regimens, as shown by a study indicating that minorities considering hyperlipidemia therapy may be less informed and less involved in the final decision-making process therefore contributing to racial disparity in health management of a nation [182].

Furthermore, while some developed societies may be made more conscious of risk factors for a given disease, heterogeneity through population migration and levels of consciousness among the different ethnic groups within a society may always change the dynamics of the situation. This indeed plays a central role in the unequal distribution of the resources contributing to disparities in the availability of health services. Most of it can be explained by the prevalence of confounders, such as lack of awareness, in which disproportionate rates seem to rank highly even in developed counties. Given the likelihood of ethnic differences in lipid profiles and the prevalence of hyperlipidemia together with the lack of research in ethnic minorities, it becomes clear that therapy of dyslipidemia remains a major concern worldwide. Being a recognizable risk factor for cardiovascular diseases, it is also questionable whether anti-lipidemic therapy attains the same effect of cardiovascular risk prevention globally under these conditions. Most importantly, profiling the gene variants in disease and drug response to anti-lipidemic therapy is the inevitable pathway towards establishing personalized treatment for this disorder. Pharmacogenetics has slowly found its rightful place in disease management. It is now well acknowledged that polymorphisms in drug-metabolizing enzymes and transporters of anti-lipidemic agents contribute to a wide variability in the pharmacokinetic response and toxicity of these drugs. In this regard, ethnicity plays an important role in defining the relevance of the genetic changes in achieving the ultimate goal of personalized drug therapy. However, as demonstrated in the preceding paragraphs, further studies are needed to explore deeper the gene-dose, gene-concentration and gene-response relationships especially for the drug metabolizing CYP450s. The more we make progress in identifying the genetic variations of dyslipidemia or drug response to therapy, the greater the likelihood that personalized medicine becomes a reality rather than remaining a myth in the foreseeable future.

Because of the uncertainties summarized above, for the time being targeted drug therapy of hyperlipidemia remains a dream of the future. Nonetheless, profiles of rare variants reflecting on the inter-individual variability in drug response are becoming more and more evident. Hence, the knowledge we have already acquired of the differential distribution of the important gene variants should provide valuable information in guiding clinicians in determining which gene variants may be relevant in screening patients for personalized therapy in clinical settings in a given society. The validity and usefulness of such an undertaking for routine procedures will depend foremost on the prevalence of such entities. Hence, recommendations for genotype-adjusted therapy will soon be of time.

4. Summary

Hypercholesterolemia is a complex disorder which presents in different forms, including the familial form, with varying underlying aetiology, and contributes substantially to CAD manifestation. Predisposing variables for the disease include modifiable risk traits, such as diet, overweight and obesity, that are controllable by adopting healthy eating habits and exercise, for example. However, diet alone is often not adequate to achieve the desired lipid lowering effect in individuals harbouring very high cholesterol levels, such as in familial hypercholesterolemia. This necessitates the use of lipid lowering medication to reduce its production or absorption or other forms of therapy including LDL apheresis or surgery. It is now well established that the response to anti-lipidemic therapy depends on genetic changes in the disease-causing as well as ADME-related genes, and the impact of these gene-drug response relationships will depend on ethnicity. Inter-ethnical variability in pharmacokinetics of anti-lipidemic agents may trigger unexpected outcomes such as therapeutic failure, adverse effects and toxicity in individuals of different ethnic origin undergoing therapy. Hence, in-depth studies on these relationships have the huge potential of achieving optimal quality use of drugs as well as improving the efficacy and safety of both prospective and currently available anti-lipidemic therapeutic agents.

Author details

Maha M. Alrasheed[1] and Nduna Dzimiri[2*]

*Address all correspondence to: dzimiri@kfshrc.edu.sa

1 Clinical Pharmacy Department, College of Pharmacy, King Saud University, Riyadh, Saudi Arabia

2 King Faisal Specialist Hospital and Research Centre, Riyadh, Saudi Arabia

References

[1] Biggerstaff KD, Wooten JS: Understanding lipoproteins as transporters of cholesterol and other lipids. *Adv Physiol Educ* 2004, 28(1–4):105–106.

[2] Durrington P: Dyslipidaemia. *Lancet* 2003, 362(9385):717–731.

[3] Carmena R, Duriez P, Fruchart JC: Atherogenic lipoprotein particles in atherosclerosis. *Circulation* 2004, 109(23 Suppl 1):III2-7.

[4] Kontush A, Chapman MJ: Antiatherogenic small, dense HDL--guardian angel of the arterial wall? *Nat Clin Pract Cardiovasc Med* 2006, 3(3):144–153.

[5] Rudkowska I, Dewailly E, Hegele RA, Boiteau V, Dube-Linteau A, Abdous B, Giguere Y, Chateau-Degat ML, Vohl MC: Gene-diet interactions on plasma lipid levels in the Inuit population. *Br J Nutr* 2013, 109(5):953–961.

[6] Bays HE, Chapman RH, Grandy S: The relationship of body mass index to diabetes mellitus, hypertension and dyslipidaemia: comparison of data from two national surveys. *Internat J Clin Prac* 2007, 61(5):737–747.

[7] Lin WY, Lee LT, Chen CY, Lo H, Hsia HH, Liu IL, Lin RS, Shau WY, Huang KC: Optimal cut-off values for obesity: using simple anthropometric indices to predict cardiovascular risk factors in Taiwan. *Int J Obes Relat Metab Disord* 2002, 26(9):1232–1238.

[8] Khoo KL, van Acker P, Defesche JC, Tan H, van de Kerkhof L, Heijnen-van Eijk SJ, Kastelein JJ, Deslypere JP: Low-density lipoprotein receptor gene mutations in a

Southeast Asian population with familial hypercholesterolemia. *Clin Genet* 2000, 58(2): 98–105.

[9] Ito MK, McGowan MP, Moriarty PM: Management of familial hypercholesterolemias in adult patients: recommendations from the National Lipid Association Expert Panel on Familial Hypercholesterolemia. *J Clin Lipidol* 2011, 5(3 Suppl):S38–S45.

[10] Medeiros AM, Alves AC, Francisco V, Bourbon M: Update of the Portuguese Familial Hypercholesterolaemia Study. *Atherosclerosis* 2010, 212(2):553–558.

[11] Vaca G, Vazquez A, Magana MT, Ramirez ML, Davalos IP, Martinez E, Marin B, Carrillo G: Mutational analysis of the LDL receptor and APOB genes in Mexican individuals with autosomal dominant hypercholesterolemia. *Atherosclerosis* 2011, 218(2):391–396.

[12] Miyake Y, Yamamura T, Sakai N, Miyata T, Kokubo Y, Yamamoto A: Update of Japanese common LDLR gene mutations and their phenotypes: mild type mutation L547V might predominate in the Japanese population. *Atherosclerosis* 2009, 203(1):153–160.

[13] Kim JH, Choi HK, Lee H, Park HY, Kim JH, Kim JW, Kim HJ, Lee ST: Novel and recurrent mutations of the LDL receptor gene in Korean patients with familial hypercholesterolemia. *Mol Cells* 2004, 18(1):63–70.

[14] Loubser O, Marais AD, Kotze MJ, Godenir N, Thiart R, Scholtz CL, de Villiers JN, Hillermann R, Firth JC, Weich HF *et al*: Founder mutations in the LDL receptor gene contribute significantly to the familial hypercholesterolemia phenotype in the indigenous South African population of mixed ancestry. *Clin Genet* 1999, 55(5):340–345.

[15] Charng MJ, Chiou KR, Chang HM, Cheng HM, Ye ZX, Lin SJ: Identification and characterization of novel low-density lipoprotein receptor mutations of familial hypercholesterolaemia patients in Taiwan. *Eur J Clin Invest* 2006, 36(12):866–874.

[16] Miyake Y, Kimura R, Kokubo Y, Okayama A, Tomoike H, Yamamura T, Miyata T: Genetic variants in PCSK9 in the Japanese population: rare genetic variants in PCSK9 might collectively contribute to plasma LDL cholesterol levels in the general population. *Atherosclerosis* 2008, 196(1):29–36.

[17] Mabuchi H, Nohara A, Noguchi T, Kobayashi J, Kawashiri MA, Inoue T, Mori M, Tada H, Nakanishi C, Yagi K *et al*: Genotypic and phenotypic features in homozygous familial hypercholesterolemia caused by proprotein convertase subtilisin/kexin type 9 (PCSK9) gain-of-function mutation. *Atherosclerosis* 2014, 236(1):54–61.

[18] Tada H, Kawashiri MA, Yoshida T, Teramoto R, Nohara A, Konno T, Inazu A, Mabuchi H, Yamagishi M, Hayashi K: Lipoprotein(a) in familial hypercholesterolemia with proprotein convertase subtilisin/kexin type 9 (PCSK9) gain-of-function mutations. *Circ J* 2016, 80(2):512–518.

[19] Shin DG, Han SM, Kim DI, Rhee MY, Lee BK, Ahn YK, Cho BR, Woo JT, Hur SH, Jeong JO *et al*: Clinical features of familial hypercholesterolemia in Korea: predictors of

pathogenic mutations and coronary artery disease - a study supported by the Korean Society of Lipidology and Atherosclerosis. *Atherosclerosis* 2015, 243(1):53–58.

[20] Abifadel M, Guerin M, Benjannet S, Rabes JP, Le Goff W, Julia Z, Hamelin J, Carreau V, Varret M, Bruckert E *et al*: Identification and characterization of new gain-of-function mutations in the PCSK9 gene responsible for autosomal dominant hypercholesterolemia. *Atherosclerosis* 2012, 223(2):394–400.

[21] Abifadel M, Varret M, Rabes JP, Allard D, Ouguerram K, Devillers M, Cruaud C, Benjannet S, Wickham L, Erlich D *et al*: Mutations in PCSK9 cause autosomal dominant hypercholesterolemia. *Nat Genet* 2003, 34(2):154–156.

[22] Timms KM, Wagner S, Samuels ME, Forbey K, Goldfine H, Jammulapati S, Skolnick MH, Hopkins PN, Hunt SC, Shattuck DM: A mutation in PCSK9 causing autosomal-dominant hypercholesterolemia in a Utah pedigree. *Hum Genet* 2004, 114(4):349–353.

[23] Leren TP: Mutations in the PCSK9 gene in Norwegian subjects with autosomal dominant hypercholesterolemia. *Clin Genet* 2004, 65(5):419–422.

[24] Wintjens R, Bozon D, Belabbas K, F MB, Girardet JP, Tounian P, Jolly M, Boccara F, Cohen A, Karsenty A *et al*: Global molecular analysis and APOE mutations in a cohort of autosomal dominant hypercholesterolemia patients in France. *J Lipid Res* 2016, 57(3): 482–491 .

[25] Rauh G, Schuster H, Schewe CK, Stratmann G, Keller C, Wolfram G, Zollner N: Independent mutation of arginine(3500) → glutamine associated with familial defective apolipoprotein B-100. *J Lipid Res* 1993, 34(5):799–805.

[26] Thomas ER, Atanur SS, Norsworthy PJ, Encheva V, Snijders AP, Game L, Vandrovcova J, Siddiq A, Seed M, Soutar AK *et al*: Identification and biochemical analysis of a novel APOB mutation that causes autosomal dominant hypercholesterolemia. *Mol Genet Genom Med* 2013, 1(3):155–161.

[27] Merino-Ibarra E, Castillo S, Mozas P, Cenarro A, Martorell E, Diaz JL, Suarez-Tembra M, Alonso R, Civeira F, Mata P *et al*: Screening of APOB gene mutations in subjects with clinical diagnosis of familial hypercholesterolemia. *Hum Biol* 2005, 77(5):663–673.

[28] Robles-Osorio L, Huerta-Zepeda A, Ordonez ML, Canizales-Quinteros S, Diaz-Villasenor A, Gutierrez-Aguilar R, Riba L, Huertas-Vazquez A, Rodriguez-Torres M, Gomez-Diaz RA *et al*: Genetic heterogeneity of autosomal dominant hypercholesterolemia in Mexico. *Arch Med Res* 2006, 37(1):102–108.

[29] Futema M, Shah S, Cooper JA, Li K, Whittall RA, Sharifi M, Goldberg O, Drogari E, Mollaki V, Wiegman A *et al*: Refinement of variant selection for the LDL cholesterol genetic risk score in the diagnosis of the polygenic form of clinical familial hypercholesterolemia and replication in samples from 6 countries. *Clin Chem* 2015, 61(1):231–238.

[30] Pimstone SN, Sun XM, du Souich C, Frohlich JJ, Hayden MR, Soutar AK: Phenotypic variation in heterozygous familial hypercholesterolemia: a comparison of Chinese

patients with the same or similar mutations in the LDL receptor gene in China or Canada. *Arterioscler Thromb Vasc Biol* 1998, 18(2):309–315.

[31] Wang J, Huff E, Janecka L, Hegele RA: Low density lipoprotein receptor (LDLR) gene mutations in Canadian subjects with familial hypercholesterolemia, but not of French descent. *Hum Mutat* 2001, 18(4):359.

[32] Roy M, Sing CF, Betard C, Davignon J: Impact of a common mutation of the LDL receptor gene, in French-Canadian patients with familial hypercholesterolemia, on means, variances and correlations among traits of lipid metabolism. *Clin Genet* 1995, 47(2):59–67.

[33] Gasparovic J, Basistova Z, Fabryova L, Wsolova L, Vohnout B, Raslova K: Familial defective apolipoprotein B-100 in Slovakia: are differences in prevalence of familial defective apolipoprotein B-100 explained by ethnicity? *Atherosclerosis* 2007, 194(2):e95–e107.

[34] Abdel-Wareth LO, Pimstone SN, Lagarde JP, Raisonnier A, Benlian P, Pritchard H, Hayden MR, Frohlich JJ: Familial defective apolipoprotein B-100 in hypercholesterolemic Chinese Canadians: identification of a unique haplotype of the apolipoprotein B-100 allele. *Atherosclerosis* 1997, 135(2):181–185.

[35] Saavedra YG, Dufour R, Davignon J, Baass A: PCSK9 R46L, lower LDL, and cardiovascular disease risk in familial hypercholesterolemia: a cross-sectional cohort study. *Arterioscler Thromb Vasc Biol* 2014, 34(12):2700–2705.

[36] Lambert G, Petrides F, Chatelais M, Blom DJ, Choque B, Tabet F, Wong G, Rye KA, Hooper AJ, Burnett JR *et al*: Elevated plasma PCSK9 level is equally detrimental for patients with nonfamilial hypercholesterolemia and heterozygous familial hypercholesterolemia, irrespective of low-density lipoprotein receptor defects. *J Am Coll Cardiol* 2014, 63(22):2365–2373.

[37] Huijgen R, Fouchier SW, Denoun M, Hutten BA, Vissers MN, Lambert G, Kastelein JJ: Plasma levels of PCSK9 and phenotypic variability in familial hypercholesterolemia. *J Lipid Res* 2012, 53(5):979–983.

[38] Gu SJ, Liu MM, Guo ZR, Wu M, Chen Q, Zhou ZY, Zhang LJ, Luo WS: Gene-gene interactions among PPARalpha/delta/gamma polymorphisms for hypertriglyceridemia in Chinese Han population. *Gene* 2013, 515(2):272–276.

[39] Tanaka T, Ordovas JM, Delgado-Lista J, Perez-Jimenez F, Marin C, Perez-Martinez P, Gomez P, Lopez-Miranda J: Peroxisome proliferator-activated receptor alpha polymorphisms and postprandial lipemia in healthy men. *J Lipid Res* 2007, 48(6): 1402–1408.

[40] Guan J, Yi H, Wu X, Su K, Tao M, Yin S: Pro12Ala polymorphism in human peroxisome proliferator activated receptor gamma is associated with hyperlipidaemia in obstructive sleep apnoea hypopnoea syndrome. *J Laryngol Otol* 2011, 125(10):1042–1048.

[41] Chen ES, Mazzotti DR, Furuya TK, Cendoroglo MS, Ramos LR, Araujo LQ, Burbano RR, Smith Mde A: Association of PPARalpha gene polymorphisms and lipid serum levels in a Brazilian elderly population. *Exp Mol Pathol* 2010, 88(1):197–201.

[42] Zietz B, Barth N, Spiegel D, Schmitz G, Scholmerich J, Schaffler A: Pro12Ala polymorphism in the peroxisome proliferator-activated receptor-gamma2 (PPARgamma2) is associated with higher levels of total cholesterol and LDL-cholesterol in male caucasian type 2 diabetes patients. *Exp Clin Endocrinol Diabetes* 2002, 110(2):60–66.

[43] Swarbrick MM, Chapman CM, McQuillan BM, Hung J, Thompson PL, Beilby JP: A Pro12Ala polymorphism in the human peroxisome proliferator-activated receptor-gamma 2 is associated with combined hyperlipidaemia in obesity. *Eur J Endocrinol* 2001, 144(3):277–282.

[44] Aberle J, Hopfer I, Beil FU, Seedorf U: Association of the T+294C polymorphism in PPAR delta with low HDL cholesterol and coronary heart disease risk in women. *Internat J Med Scie* 2006, 3(3):108–111.

[45] Skogsberg J, McMahon AD, Karpe F, Hamsten A, Packard CJ, Ehrenborg E: Peroxisome proliferator activated receptor delta genotype in relation to cardiovascular risk factors and risk of coronary heart disease in hypercholesterolaemic men. *J Intern Med* 2003, 254(6):597–604.

[46] Thompson JF, Lira ME, Durham LK, Clark RW, Bamberger MJ, Milos PM: Polymorphisms in the CETP gene and association with CETP mass and HDL levels. *Atherosclerosis* 2003, 167(2):195–204.

[47] Park KW, Choi JH, Kim HK, Oh S, Chae IH, Kim HS, Oh BH, Lee MM, Park YB, Choi YS: The association of cholesteryl ester transfer protein polymorphism with high-density lipoprotein cholesterol and coronary artery disease in Koreans. *Clin Genet* 2003, 63(1):31–38.

[48] Weissglas-Volkov D, Aguilar-Salinas CA, Nikkola E, Deere KA, Cruz-Bautista I, Arellano-Campos O, Munoz-Hernandez LL, Gomez-Munguia L, Ordonez-Sanchez ML, Reddy PM *et al*: Genomic study in Mexicans identifies a new locus for triglycerides and refines European lipid loci. *J Med Genet* 2013, 50(5):298–308.

[49] Tada H, Kawashiri MA, Ohtani R, Noguchi T, Nakanishi C, Konno T, Hayashi K, Nohara A, Inazu A, Kobayashi J *et al*: A novel type of familial hypercholesterolemia: double heterozygous mutations in LDL receptor and LDL receptor adaptor protein 1 gene. *Atherosclerosis* 2011, 219(2):663–666.

[50] Filigheddu F, Quagliarini F, Campagna F, Secci T, Degortes S, Zaninello R, Argiolas G, Verna R, Pitzoi S, Frau F *et al*: Prevalence and clinical features of heterozygous carriers of autosomal recessive hypercholesterolemia in Sardinia. *Atherosclerosis* 2009, 207(1): 162–167.

[51] Canizales-Quinteros S, Aguilar-Salinas CA, Huertas-Vazquez A, Ordonez-Sanchez ML, Rodriguez-Torres M, Venturas-Gallegos JL, Riba L, Ramirez-Jimenez S, Salas-

Montiel R, Medina-Palacios G *et al*: A novel ARH splice site mutation in a Mexican kindred with autosomal recessive hypercholesterolemia. *Hum Genet* 2005, 116(1–2): 114–120.

[52] Barbagallo CM, Emmanuele G, Cefalu AB, Fiore B, Noto D, Mazzarino MC, Pace A, Brogna A, Rizzo M, Corsini A *et al*: Autosomal recessive hypercholesterolemia in a Sicilian kindred harboring the 432insA mutation of the ARH gene. *Atherosclerosis* 2003, 166(2):395–400.

[53] Weissglas-Volkov D, Aguilar-Salinas CA, Sinsheimer JS, Riba L, Huertas-Vazquez A, Ordonez-Sanchez ML, Rodriguez-Guillen R, Cantor RM, Tusie-Luna T, Pajukanta P: Investigation of variants identified in caucasian genome-wide association studies for plasma high-density lipoprotein cholesterol and triglycerides levels in Mexican dyslipidemic study samples. *Circ Cardiovasc Genet* 2010, 3(1):31–38.

[54] Li YY, Wu XY, Xu J, Qian Y, Zhou CW, Wang B: Apo A5 -1131T/C, FgB -455G/A, −148C/T, and CETP TaqIB gene polymorphisms and coronary artery disease in the Chinese population: a meta-analysis of 15,055 subjects. *Mol Biol Rep* 2013, 40(2):1997–2014.

[55] Utermann G: Apolipoproteins, quantitative lipoprotein traits and multifactorial hyperlipidaemia. *Ciba Foundation Symp* 1987, 130:52–69.

[56] Rodriguez CJ, Daviglus ML, Swett K, Gonzalez HM, Gallo LC, Wassertheil-Smoller S, Giachello AL, Teng Y, Schneiderman N, Talavera GA *et al*: Dyslipidemia patterns among Hispanics/Latinos of diverse background in the United States. *Am J Med* 2014, 127(12): 1186–1194, e1181.

[57] Basu A, Tang H, Lewis CE, North K, Curb JD, Quertermous T, Mosley TH, Boerwinkle E, Zhu X, Risch NJ: Admixture mapping of quantitative trait loci for blood lipids in African-Americans. *Hum Mol Genet* 2009, 18(11):2091–2098.

[58] Paramsothy P, Knopp R, Bertoni AG, Tsai MY, Rue T, Heckbert SR: Combined hyperlipidemia in relation to race/ethnicity, obesity, and insulin resistance in the Multi-Ethnic Study of Atherosclerosis (MESA). *Metabolism* 2009, 58(2):212–219.

[59] Lu Y, Tayebi N, Li H, Saha N, Yang H, Heng CK: Association of CETP Taq1B and -629C > A polymorphisms with coronary artery disease and lipid levels in the multi-ethnic Singaporean population. *Lipids Health Dis* 2013, 12:85.

[60] Li D, Zhang GL, Lou YQ, Li Q, Wang X, Bu XY: Genetic polymorphisms in MDR1 and CYP3A5 and MDR1 haplotype in mainland Chinese Han, Uygur and Kazakh ethnic groups. *J Clin Pharmac Ther* 2007, 32(1):89–95.

[61] Deo RC, Reich D, Tandon A, Akylbekova E, Patterson N, Waliszewska A, Kathiresan S, Sarpong D, Taylor HA, Jr., Wilson JG: Genetic differences between the determinants of lipid profile phenotypes in African and European Americans: the Jackson Heart Study. *PLoS Genet* 2009, 5(1):e1000342.

[62] WHO: Obesity: preventing and managing the global epidemic. Report of a WHO consultation. *WHO Tech Rep Ser* 2000, 894:i–xii, 1–253.

[63] Consortium WHOE: Appropriate body-mass index for Asian populations and its implications for policy and intervention strategies. *Lancet* 2004, 363(9403):157–163.

[64] Swinburn BA, Ley SJ, Carmichael HE, Plank LD: Body size and composition in Polynesians. *Int J Obes Relat Metab Disord* 1999, 23(11):1178–1183.

[65] Consortium WE: Obesity and overweight. *http://wwwwhoint/mediacentre/factsheets/fs311/en/#* 2013, Fact sheet N°311; Updated March 2013.

[66] Deurenberg P, Yap M, van Staveren WA: Body mass index and percent body fat: a meta-analysis among different ethnic groups. *Int J Obes Relat Metab Disord* 1998, 22(12):1164–1171.

[67] Hu FB, Wang B, Chen C, Jin Y, Yang J, Stampfer MJ, Xu X: Body mass index and cardiovascular risk factors in a rural Chinese population. *Am J Epidemiol* 2000, 151(1): 88–97.

[68] Deurenberg-Yap M, Chew SK, Deurenberg P: Elevated body fat percentage and cardiovascular risks at low body mass index levels among Singaporean Chinese, Malays and Indians. *Obesity Rev* 2002, 3(3):209–215.

[69] Wen CP, David Cheng TY, Tsai SP, Chan HT, Hsu HL, Hsu CC, Eriksen MP: Are Asians at greater mortality risks for being overweight than Caucasians? Redefining obesity for Asians. *Public Health Nutr* 2009, 12(4):497–506.

[70] Wulan SN, Westerterp KR, Plasqui G: Ethnic differences in body composition and the associated metabolic profile: a comparative study between Asians and Caucasians. *Maturitas* 2010, 65(4):315–319.

[71] Goldstein KM, Melnyk SD, Zullig LL, Stechuchak KM, Oddone E, Bastian LA, Rakley S, Olsen MK, Bosworth HB: Heart matters: gender and racial differences cardiovascular disease risk factor control among veterans. *Women's Health Issues* 2014, 24(5):477–483.

[72] Liao PJ, Xie RB, Yin RX, Wei DX, Huang J, Huang F, Li H, Lin WX, Wu JZ, Pan SL: Serum lipid profiles, the prevalence of dyslipidemia and the risk factors in two isolated Chinese minorities. *Intl J Clin Experiment Med* 2015, 8(10):19200–19211.

[73] Phipps ME, Chan KK, Naidu R, Mohamad NW, Hoh BP, Quek KF, Ahmad B, Harnida SM, Zain AZ, Kadir KA: Cardio-metabolic health risks in indigenous populations of Southeast Asia and the influence of urbanization. *BMC Public Health* 2015, 15:47.

[74] Shammas NW, Kapalis MJ, Deckert J, Harris M, Dippel EJ, Labroo A, McKinney D: Effectiveness of statin-gemfibrozil combination therapy in patients with mixed hyperlipidemia: experience of a community lipid clinic and safety review from the literature. *Prevent Cardiol* 2003, 6(4):189–194.

[75] Christidis DS, Liberopoulos EN, Kakafika AI, Miltiadous GA, Cariolou M, Ganotakis ES, Mikhailidis DP, Elisaf MS: The effect of apolipoprotein E polymorphism on the response to lipid-lowering treatment with atorvastatin or fenofibrate. *J Cardiovasc Pharmacol Ther* 2006, 11(3):211–221.

[76] Chen Q, Zhang T, Wang JF, Wei DQ: Advances in human cytochrome p450 and personalized medicine. *Curr Drug Metab* 2011, 12(5):436–444.

[77] Cheng JW, Frishman WH, Aronow WS: Updates on cytochrome P450-mediated cardiovascular drug interactions. *Am J Ther* 2009, 16(2):155–163.

[78] Scandlyn MJ, Stuart EC, Rosengren RJ: Sex-specific differences in CYP450 isoforms in humans. *Expert Opin Drug Metab Toxicol* 2008, 4(4):413–424.

[79] Pilgrim JL, Gerostamoulos D, Drummer OH: Review: pharmacogenetic aspects of the effect of cytochrome P450 polymorphisms on serotonergic drug metabolism, response, interactions, and adverse effects. *Forensic Sci Med Path* 2011, 7(2):162–184.

[80] Kohrle J: Thyroid hormone transporters in health and disease: advances in thyroid hormone deiodination. *Best Pract Res* 2007, 21(2):173–191.

[81] Goldstein JA: Clinical relevance of genetic polymorphisms in the human CYP2C subfamily. *Br J Clin Pharmacol* 2001, 52(4):349–355.

[82] Goldstein JA, de Morais SM: Biochemistry and molecular biology of the human CYP2C subfamily. *Pharmacogenetics* 1994, 4(6):285–299.

[83] Lee CR, Goldstein JA, Pieper JA: Cytochrome P450 2C9 polymorphisms: a comprehensive review of the in-vitro and human data. *Pharmacogenetics* 2002, 12(3):251–263.

[84] Kirchheiner J, Brockmoller J: Clinical consequences of cytochrome P450 2C9 polymorphisms. *Clin Pharmacol Ther* 2005, 77(1):1–16.

[85] Kirchheiner J, Kudlicz D, Meisel C, Bauer S, Meineke I, Roots I, Brockmoller J: Influence of CYP2C9 polymorphisms on the pharmacokinetics and cholesterol-lowering activity of (−)-3S,5R-fluvastatin and (+)-3R,5S-fluvastatin in healthy volunteers. *Clin Pharmacol Ther* 2003, 74(2):186–194.

[86] Thomas FJ, McLeod HL, Watters JW: Pharmacogenomics: the influence of genomic variation on drug response. *Curr Top Med Chem* 2004, 4(13):1399–1409.

[87] Grarup N, Andersen MK, Andreasen CH, Albrechtsen A, Borch-Johnsen K, Jorgensen T, Auwerx J, Schmitz O, Hansen T, Pedersen O: Studies of the common DIO2 Thr92Ala polymorphism and metabolic phenotypes in 7342 Danish white subjects. *J Clin Endocrinol Metab* 2007, 92(1):363–366.

[88] Ingelman-Sundberg M, Oscarson M, McLellan RA: Polymorphic human cytochrome P450 enzymes: an opportunity for individualized drug treatment. *Trend Pharmacol Sci* 1999, 20(8):342–349.

[89] Mihaljevic-Peles A, Sagud M, Bozina N, Zivkovic M, Jovanovic N: Pharmacogenetics and antipsychotics in the light of personalized pharmacotherapy. *Psychiatria Danubina* 2010, 22(2):335–337.

[90] Shahrokh K, Cheatham TE, 3rd, Yost GS: Conformational dynamics of CYP3A4 demonstrate the important role of Arg212 coupled with the opening of ingress, egress and solvent channels to dehydrogenation of 4-hydroxy-tamoxifen. *Biochim Biophys Acta* 2012, 1820(10):1605–1617.

[91] Schelleman H, Limdi NA, Kimmel SE: Ethnic differences in warfarin maintenance dose requirement and its relationship with genetics. *Pharmacogenomics* 2008, 9(9): 1331–1346.

[92] Muszkat M: Interethnic differences in drug response: the contribution of genetic variability in beta adrenergic receptor and cytochrome P4502C9. *Clin Pharmacol Ther* 2007, 82(2):215–218.

[93] McGraw J, Waller D: Cytochrome P450 variations in different ethnic populations. *Expert Opin Drug Metab Toxicol* 2012, 8(3):371–382.

[94] Jaja C, Burke W, Thummel K, Edwards K, Veenstra DL: Cytochrome p450 enzyme polymorphism frequency in indigenous and native american populations: a systematic review. *Commun Genet* 2008, 11(3):141–149.

[95] Kurose K, Sugiyama E, Saito Y: Population differences in major functional polymorphisms of pharmacokinetics/pharmacodynamics-related genes in Eastern Asians and Europeans: implications in the clinical trials for novel drug development. *Drug Metab Pharmacokinet* 2012, 27(1):9–54.

[96] Jazdzewski K, Boguslawska J, Jendrzejewski J, Liyanarachchi S, Pachucki J, Wardyn KA, Nauman A, de la Chapelle A: Thyroid hormone receptor beta (THRB) is a major target gene for microRNAs deregulated in papillary thyroid carcinoma (PTC). *J Clin Endocrinol Metab* 2011, 96(3):E546–E553.

[97] Polimanti R, Piacentini S, Manfellotto D, Fuciarelli M: Human genetic variation of CYP450 superfamily: analysis of functional diversity in worldwide populations. *Pharmacogenomics* 2012, 13(16):1951–1960.

[98] Goldstein JA, Ishizaki T, Chiba K, de Morais SM, Bell D, Krahn PM, Evans DA: Frequencies of the defective CYP2C19 alleles responsible for the mephenytoin poor metabolizer phenotype in various Oriental, Caucasian, Saudi Arabian and American black populations. *Pharmacogenetics* 1997, 7(1):59–64.

[99] Man M, Farmen M, Dumaual C, Teng CH, Moser B, Irie S, Noh GJ, Njau R, Close S, Wise S *et al*: Genetic variation in metabolizing enzyme and transporter genes: comprehensive assessment in 3 major East Asian subpopulations with comparison to Caucasians and Africans. *J Clin Pharmacol* 2010, 50(8): 929–940.

[100] Luo HR, Poland RE, Lin KM, Wan YJ: Genetic polymorphism of cytochrome P450 2C19 in Mexican Americans: a cross-ethnic comparative study. *Clin Pharmacol Ther* 2006, 80(1):33–40.

[101] Zuo LJ, Guo T, Xia DY, Jia LH: Allele and genotype frequencies of CYP3A4, CYP2C19, and CYP2D6 in Han, Uighur, Hui, and Mongolian Chinese populations. *Genet Test Mol Biomarkers* 2012, 16(2):102–108.

[102] Li Y, Yang H, Zou X, Xiong L, Li Z, Luo J, Zhao B, Liu W, Du X: Analysis of the CYP2C19 genetic polymorphism in Han and Uyghur patients with cardiovascular and cerebrovascular diseases in the Kashi area of Xinjiang. *Med Sci Monit* 2014, 20:2213–2218.

[103] Yin SJ, Ni YB, Wang SM, Wang X, Lou YQ, Zhang GL: Differences in genotype and allele frequency distributions of polymorphic drug metabolizing enzymes CYP2C19 and CYP2D6 in mainland Chinese Mongolian, Hui and Han populations. *J Clin Pharm Ther* 2012, 37(3):364–369.

[104] Chan SL, Samaranayake N, Ross CJ, Toh MT, Carleton B, Hayden MR, Teo YY, Dissanayake VH, Brunham LR: Genetic diversity of variants involved in drug response and metabolism in Sri Lankan populations: implications for clinical implementation of pharmacogenomics. *Pharmacogenet Genom* 2016, 26(1):28–39.

[105] Sipeky C, Weber A, Szabo M, Melegh BI, Janicsek I, Tarlos G, Szabo I, Sumegi K, Melegh B: High prevalence of CYP2C19*2 allele in Roma samples: study on Roma and Hungarian population samples with review of the literature. *Mol Biol Rep* 2013, 40(8):4727–4735.

[106] Strom CM, Goos D, Crossley B, Zhang K, Buller-Burkle A, Jarvis M, Quan F, Peng M, Sun W: Testing for variants in CYP2C19: population frequencies and testing experience in a clinical laboratory. *Genet Med* 2012, 14(1):95–100.

[107] Daly AK: Pharmacogenetics of drug metabolizing enzymes in the United Kingdom population: review of current knowledge and comparison with selected European populations. *Drug Metabol Personalized Ther* 2015, 30(3):165–174.

[108] Fricke-Galindo I, Cespedes-Garro C, Rodrigues-Soares F, Naranjo ME, Delgado A, de Andres F, Lopez-Lopez M, Penas-Lledo E, A LL: Interethnic variation of CYP2C19 alleles, 'predicted' phenotypes and 'measured' metabolic phenotypes across world populations. *Pharmacogenomics J* 2016, 16(2):113–123.

[109] Barter ZE, Tucker GT, Rowland-Yeo K: Differences in cytochrome p450-mediated pharmacokinetics between Chinese and Caucasian populations predicted by mechanistic physiologically based pharmacokinetic modelling. *Clin Pharmacokinet* 2013, 52(12):1085–1100.

[110] Pang YS, Wong LP, Lee TC, Mustafa AM, Mohamed Z, Lang CC: Genetic polymorphism of cytochrome P450 2C19 in healthy Malaysian subjects. *Br J Clin Pharmacol* 2004, 58(3): 332–335.

[111] Zhou SF, Di YM, Chan E, Du YM, Chow VD, Xue CC, Lai X, Wang JC, Li CG, Tian M *et al*: Clinical pharmacogenetics and potential application in personalized medicine. *Curr Drug Metab* 2008, 9(8):738–784.

[112] Ramsjo M, Aklillu E, Bohman L, Ingelman-Sundberg M, Roh HK, Bertilsson L: CYP2C19 activity comparison between Swedes and Koreans: effect of genotype, sex, oral contraceptive use, and smoking. *Eur J Clin Pharmacol* 2010, 66(9):871–877.

[113] Cespedes-Garro C, Fricke-Galindo I, Naranjo ME, Rodrigues-Soares F, Farinas H, de Andres F, Lopez-Lopez M, Penas-Lledo EM, A LL: Worldwide interethnic variability and geographical distribution of CYP2C9 genotypes and phenotypes. *Expert Opin Drug Metab Toxicol* 2015, 11(12):1893–1905.

[114] Hatta FH, Lundblad M, Ramsjo M, Kang JH, Roh HK, Bertilsson L, Eliasson E, Aklillu E: Differences in CYP2C9 genotype and enzyme activity between Swedes and Koreans of relevance for personalized medicine: role of ethnicity, genotype, smoking, age, and sex. *OMICS* 2015, 19(6):346–353.

[115] Schwarz UI: Clinical relevance of genetic polymorphisms in the human CYP2C9 gene. *Eur J Clin Invest* 2003, 33(Suppl 2):23–30.

[116] LLerena A, Dorado P, O'Kirwan F, Jepson R, Licinio J, Wong ML: Lower frequency of CYP2C9*2 in Mexican-Americans compared to Spaniards. *Pharmacogenomics J* 2004, 4(6):403–406.

[117] Allabi AC, Gala JL, Desager JP, Heusterspreute M, Horsmans Y: Genetic polymorphisms of CYP2C9 and CYP2C19 in the Beninese and Belgian populations. *Br J Clin Pharmacol* 2003, 56(6):653–657.

[118] Scordo MG, Aklillu E, Yasar U, Dahl ML, Spina E, Ingelman-Sundberg M: Genetic polymorphism of cytochrome P450 2C9 in a Caucasian and a black African population. *Br J Clin Pharmacol* 2001, 52(4):447–450.

[119] Sosa-Macias M, Lazalde-Ramos BP, Galaviz-Hernandez C, Rangel-Villalobos H, Salazar-Flores J, Martinez-Sevilla VM, Martinez-Fierro ML, Dorado P, Wong ML, Licinio J *et al*: Influence of admixture components on CYP2C9*2 allele frequency in eight indigenous populations from Northwest Mexico. *Pharmacogenomics J* 2013, 13(6):567–572.

[120] Hashemi-Soteh SM, Shahabi-Majd N, Gholizadeh AR, Shiran MR: Allele and genotype frequencies of CYP2C9 within an Iranian population (Mazandaran). *Genet Test Mol Biomarkers* 2012, 16(7):817–821.

[121] Sipeky C, Lakner L, Szabo M, Takacs I, Tamasi V, Polgar N, Falus A, Melegh B: Interethnic differences of CYP2C9 alleles in healthy Hungarian and Roma population samples: relationship to worldwide allelic frequencies. *Blood Cell Mol Dis* 2009, 43(3): 239–242.

[122] Nakai K, Habano W, Nakai K, Fukushima N, Suwabe A, Moriya S, Osano K, Gurwitz D: Ethnic differences in CYP2C9*2 (Arg144Cys) and CYP2C9*3 (Ile359Leu) genotypes in Japanese and Israeli populations. *Life Sci* 2005, 78(1):107–111.

[123] Castelan-Martinez OD, Hoyo-Vadillo C, Sandoval-Garcia E, Sandoval-Ramirez L, Gonzalez-Ibarra M, Solano-Solano G, Gomez-Diaz RA, Parra EJ, Cruz M, Valladares-Salgado A: Allele frequency distribution of CYP2C9 2 and CYP2C9 3 polymorphisms in six Mexican populations. *Gene* 2013, 523(2):167–172.

[124] Dorado P, Sosa-Macias MG, Penas-Lledo EM, Alanis-Banuelos RE, Wong ML, Licinio J, Lares-Asseff I, Llerena A: CYP2C9 allele frequency differences between populations of Mexican-Mestizo, Mexican-Tepehuano, and Spaniards. *Pharmacogenomics J* 2011, 11(2):108–112.

[125] Motshoge T, Tawe L, Muthoga CW, Allotey J, Romano R, Quaye I, Paganotti GM: Cytochrome P450 2C8*2 allele in Botswana: Human genetic diversity and public health implications. *Acta tropica* 2016, 157:54–58.

[126] Garcia-Martin E, Martinez C, Ladero JM, Agundez JA: Interethnic and intraethnic variability of CYP2C8 and CYP2C9 polymorphisms in healthy individuals. *Mol Diagnosis Ther* 2006, 10(1):29–40.

[127] Wu X, Zuo J, Guo T, Yuan L: CYP2C8 polymorphism frequencies among Han, Uighur, Hui, and Mongolian Chinese populations. *Genet Test Mol Biomarkers* 2013, 17(2):104–108.

[128] Arun Kumar AS, Chakradhara Rao US, Umamaheswaran G, Ramu P, Kesavan R, Shewade DG, Balachandar J, Adithan C: Haplotype structures of common variants of CYP2C8, CYP2C9, and ADRB1 genes in a South Indian population. *Genet Test Mol Biomarkers* 2011, 15(6):407–413.

[129] Kudzi W, Dodoo AN, Mills JJ: Characterisation of CYP2C8, CYP2C9 and CYP2C19 polymorphisms in a Ghanaian population. *BMC Med Genet* 2009, 10:124.

[130] Kim JH, Cheong HS, Park BL, Kim LH, Shin HJ, Na HS, Chung MW, Shin HD: Direct sequencing and comprehensive screening of genetic polymorphisms on CYP2 family genes (CYP2A6, CYP2B6, CYP2C8, and CYP2E1) in five ethnic populations. *Arch Pharm Res* 2015, 38(1):115–128.

[131] Britzi M, Bialer M, Arcavi L, Shachbari A, Kapitulnik T, Soback S: Genetic polymorphism of CYP2D6 and CYP2C19 metabolism determined by phenotyping Israeli ethnic groups. *Ther Drug Monit* 2000, 22(5):510–516.

[132] Jin TB, Ma LF, Zhang JY, Yuan DY, Sun Q, Zong TY, Geng TT, Cui YL, Kang LL, Chen C: Polymorphisms and phenotypic analysis of cytochrome P450 2D6 in the Tibetan population. *Gene* 2013, 527(1):360–365.

[133] Griman P, Moran Y, Valero G, Loreto M, Borjas L, Chiurillo MA: CYP2D6 gene variants in urban/admixed and Amerindian populations of Venezuela: pharmacogenetics and anthropological implications. *Annal Hum Biol* 2012, 39(2):137–142.

[134] Xie HG, Stein CM, Kim RB, Wilkinson GR, Flockhart DA, Wood AJ: Allelic, genotypic and phenotypic distributions of S-mephenytoin 4'-hydroxylase (CYP2C19) in healthy Caucasian populations of European descent throughout the world. *Pharmacogenetics* 1999, 9(5):539–549.

[135] Mendoza R, Wan YJ, Poland RE, Smith M, Zheng Y, Berman N, Lin KM: CYP2D6 polymorphism in a Mexican American population. *Clin Pharmacol Ther* 2001, 70(6):552–560.

[136] Luo HR, Aloumanis V, Lin KM, Gurwitz D, Wan YJ: Polymorphisms of CYP2C19 and CYP2D6 in Israeli ethnic groups. *Am J Pharmacogenomics* 2004, 4(6):395–401.

[137] Scordo MG, Caputi AP, D'Arrigo C, Fava G, Spina E: Allele and genotype frequencies of CYP2C9, CYP2C19 and CYP2D6 in an Italian population. *Pharmacol Res* 2004, 50(2): 195–200.

[138] Cespedes-Garro C, Jimenez-Arce G, Naranjo ME, Barrantes R, Llerena A: Ethnic background and CYP2D6 genetic polymorphisms in Costa Ricans. *Revista Biol Tropical* 2014, 62(4):1659–1671.

[139] Serpe L, Canaparo R, Scordo MG, Spina E: Pharmacogenetics of drug-metabolizing enzymes in Italian populations. *Drug Metabol Personalized Ther* 2015, 30(2):107–120.

[140] Riccardi LN, Lanzellotto R, Luiselli D, Ceccardi S, Falconi M, Bini C, Pelotti S: CYP2D6 genotyping in natives and immigrants from the Emilia-Romagna Region (Italy). *Genet Test Mol Biomarkers* 2011, 15(11):801–806.

[141] Gaedigk A, Isidoro-Garcia M, Pearce RE, Sanchez S, Garcia-Solaesa V, Lorenzo-Romo C, Gonzalez-Tejera G, Corey S: Discovery of the nonfunctional CYP2D6 31 allele in Spanish, Puerto Rican, and US Hispanic populations. *Eur J Clin Pharmacol* 2010, 66(9): 859–864.

[142] Leathart JB, London SJ, Steward A, Adams JD, Idle JR, Daly AK: CYP2D6 phenotype-genotype relationships in African-Americans and Caucasians in Los Angeles. *Pharmacogenetics* 1998, 8(6):529–541.

[143] Fluck CE, Mullis PE, Pandey AV: Reduction in hepatic drug metabolizing CYP3A4 activities caused by P450 oxidoreductase mutations identified in patients with disordered steroid metabolism. *Biochem Biophys Res Commun* 2010, 401(1):149–153.

[144] Keshava C, McCanlies EC, Weston A: CYP3A4 polymorphisms--potential risk factors for breast and prostate cancer: a HuGE review. *Am J Epidemiol* 2004, 160(9):825–841.

[145] Lai Y, Zhang J, Wang YX, Wang XD, Li JL, Wang YH, Zeng YJ, Huang M: CYP3A5*3 and MDR-1 C3435T single nucleotide polymorphisms in six Chinese ethnic groups. *Pharmazie* 2011, 66(2):136–140.

[146] Kohlrausch FB, Carracedo A, Hutz MH: Characterization of CYP1A2, CYP2C19, CYP3A4 and CYP3A5 polymorphisms in South Brazilians. *Mol Biol Rep* 2014, 41(3): 1453–1460.

[147] Suarez-Kurtz G, Vargens DD, Santoro AB, Hutz MH, de Moraes ME, Pena SD, Ribeiro-dos-Santos A, Romano-Silva MA, Struchiner CJ: Global pharmacogenomics: distribution of CYP3A5 polymorphisms and phenotypes in the Brazilian population. *PLoS One* 2014, 9(1):e83472.

[148] Bigos KL, Bies RR, Pollock BG, Lowy JJ, Zhang F, Weinberger DR: Genetic variation in CYP3A43 explains racial difference in olanzapine clearance. *Mol Psychiatry* 2011, 16(6): 620–625.

[149] McDaniel DO, Thurber T, Lewis-Traylor A, Berry C, Barber WH, Zhou X, Bigler S, Vance R: Differential association of cytochrome P450 3A4 genotypes with onsets of breast tumors in African American versus Caucasian patients. *J Investig Med* 2011, 59(7):1096–1103.

[150] Chowbay B, Zhou S, Lee EJ: An interethnic comparison of polymorphisms of the genes encoding drug-metabolizing enzymes and drug transporters: experience in Singapore. *Drug Metab Rev* 2005, 37(2):327–378.

[151] Balram C, Zhou Q, Cheung YB, Lee EJ: CYP3A5*3 and *6 single nucleotide polymorphisms in three distinct Asian populations. *Eur J Clin Pharmacol* 2003, 59(2):123–126.

[152] Qi GZ, Zhang ZY, Wang X, Yin SJ, Lou YQ, Zhang GL: Functional allele and genotype frequencies of CYP1A2, CYP2B6 and iNOS among mainland Chinese Tibetan, Mongolian, Uygur and Han populations. *J Clin Pharm Ther* 2016, 41(1):84–91.

[153] Szalai R, Magyari L, Matyas P, Duga B, Banfai Z, Szabo A, Kovesdi E, Melegh B: Genetic polymorphisms in promoter and intronic regions of CYP1A2 gene in Roma and Hungarian population samples. *Environ Toxicol Pharmacol* 2014, 38(3):814–820.

[154] Sosa-Macias M, Llerena A: Cytochrome P450 genetic polymorphisms of Mexican indigenous populations. *Drug Metabol Drug Interact* 2013, 28(4):193–208.

[155] Lim JS, Singh O, Ramasamy RD, Ramasamy S, Subramanian K, Lee EJ, Chowbay B: Pharmacogenetics of CYP1A2, novel polymorphisms and haplotypes in three distinct Asian populations. *Drug Metabol Pharmacokinet* 2010, 25(6):616–623.

[156] Aitchison KJ, Gonzalez FJ, Quattrochi LC, Sapone A, Zhao JH, Zaher H, Elizondo G, Bryant C, Munro J, Collier DA *et al*: Identification of novel polymorphisms in the 5′ flanking region of CYP1A2, characterization of interethnic variability, and investigation of their functional significance. *Pharmacogenetics* 2000, 10(8):695–704.

[157] Bailon-Soto CE, Galaviz-Hernandez C, Lazalde-Ramos BP, Hernandez-Velazquez D, Salas-Pacheco J, Lares-Assef I, Sosa-Macias M: Influence of CYP1A1*2C on high triglyceride levels in female Mexican indigenous Tarahumaras. *Arch Med Res* 2014, 45(5):409–416.

[158] Klimentidis YC, Wineinger NE, Vazquez AI, de Los Campos G: Multiple metabolic genetic risk scores and type 2 diabetes risk in three racial/ethnic groups. *J Clin Endocrinol Metab* 2014, 99(9):E1814–E1818.

[159] Garte SJ, Trachman J, Crofts F, Toniolo P, Buxbaum J, Bayo S, Taioli E: Distribution of composite CYP1A1 genotypes in Africans, African-Americans and Caucasians. *Hum Hered* 1996, 46(3):121–127.

[160] Zhang A, Xing Q, Qin S, Du J, Wang L, Yu L, Li X, Xu L, Xu M, Feng G *et al*: Intra-ethnic differences in genetic variants of the UGT-glucuronosyltransferase 1A1 gene in Chinese populations. *Pharmacogenomics J* 2007, 7(5):333–338.

[161] Lampe JW, Bigler J, Horner NK, Potter JD: UDP-glucuronosyltransferase (UGT1A1*28 and UGT1A6*2) polymorphisms in Caucasians and Asians: relationships to serum bilirubin concentrations. *Pharmacogenetics* 1999, 9(3):341–349.

[162] Fohner A, Muzquiz LI, Austin MA, Gaedigk A, Gordon A, Thornton T, Rieder MJ, Pershouse MA, Putnam EA, Howlett K *et al*: Pharmacogenetics in American Indian populations: analysis of CYP2D6, CYP3A4, CYP3A5, and CYP2C9 in the Confederated Salish and Kootenai Tribes. *Pharmacogenet Genomics* 2013, 23(8):403–414.

[163] Marusic S, Lisicic A, Horvatic I, Bacic-Vrca V, Bozina N: Atorvastatin-related rhabdomyolysis and acute renal failure in a genetically predisposed patient with potential drug-drug interaction. *Internat J Clin Pharm* 2012, 34(6):825–827.

[164] Riedmaier S, Klein K, Hofmann U, Keskitalo JE, Neuvonen PJ, Schwab M, Niemi M, Zanger UM: UDP-glucuronosyltransferase (UGT) polymorphisms affect atorvastatin lactonization in vitro and in vivo. *Clin Pharmacol Ther* 2010, 87(1):65–73.

[165] Cho SK, Oh ES, Park K, Park MS, Chung JY: The UGT1A3*2 polymorphism affects atorvastatin lactonization and lipid-lowering effect in healthy volunteers. *Pharmacogenet Genomics* 2012, 22(8):598–605.

[166] Stormo C, Bogsrud MP, Hermann M, Asberg A, Piehler AP, Retterstol K, Kringen MK: UGT1A1*28 is associated with decreased systemic exposure of atorvastatin lactone. *Mol Diagnos Ther* 2013, 17(4):233–237.

[167] Bae JW, Choi CI, Lee JH, Jang CG, Chung MW, Lee SY: Effects of UDP-glucuronosyltransferase polymorphisms on the pharmacokinetics of ezetimibe in healthy subjects. *Eur J Clin Pharmacol* 2011, 67(1):39–45.

[168] Kolovou G, Kolovou V, Mihas C, Giannakopoulou V, Vasiliadis I, Boussoula E, Kollia A, Boutsikou M, Katsiki N, Mavrogeni S: Cholesteryl ester transfer protein and ATP-

binding cassette transporter A1 genotype alter the atorvastatin and simvastatin efficacy: time for genotype-guided therapy? *Angiology* 2013, 64(4):266–272.

[169] Anagnostopoulou K, Kolovou G, Kostakou P, Mihas C, Mikhailidis D, Cokkinos DV: Pharmacogenetic study of cholesteryl ester transfer protein gene and simvastatin treatment in hypercholesterolaemic subjects. *Expert Opin Pharmacother* 2007, 8(15): 2459–2463.

[170] DeGorter MK, Tirona RG, Schwarz UI, Choi YH, Dresser GK, Suskin N, Myers K, Zou G, Iwuchukwu O, Wei WQ *et al*: Clinical and pharmacogenetic predictors of circulating atorvastatin and rosuvastatin concentrations in routine clinical care. *Circ Cardiovasc Genet* 2013, 6(4):400–408.

[171] Fu Q, Li YP, Gao Y, Yang SH, Lu PQ, Jia M, Zhang LR: Lack of association between SLCO1B1 polymorphism and the lipid-lowering effects of atorvastatin and simvastatin in Chinese individuals. *Eur J Clin Pharmacol* 2013, 69(6):1269–1274.

[172] Voora D, Shah SH, Spasojevic I, Ali S, Reed CR, Salisbury BA, Ginsburg GS: The SLCO1B1*5 genetic variant is associated with statin-induced side effects. *J Am Coll Cardiol* 2009, 54(17):1609–1616.

[173] Oswald S, Konig J, Lutjohann D, Giessmann T, Kroemer HK, Rimmbach C, Rosskopf D, Fromm MF, Siegmund W: Disposition of ezetimibe is influenced by polymorphisms of the hepatic uptake carrier OATP1B1. *Pharmacogenet Genomics* 2008, 18(7):559–568.

[174] Bercovich D, Friedlander Y, Korem S, Houminer A, Hoffman A, Kleinberg L, Shochat C, Leitersdorf E, Meiner V: The association of common SNPs and haplotypes in the CETP and MDR1 genes with lipids response to fluvastatin in familial hypercholesterolemia. *Atherosclerosis* 2006, 185(1):97–107.

[175] Miltiadous G, Xenophontos S, Bairaktari E, Ganotakis M, Cariolou M, Elisaf M: Genetic and environmental factors affecting the response to statin therapy in patients with molecularly defined familial hypercholesterolaemia. *Pharmacogenet Genomics* 2005, 15(4):219–225.

[176] Chasman DI, Posada D, Subrahmanyan L, Cook NR, Stanton VP, Jr., Ridker PM: Pharmacogenetic study of statin therapy and cholesterol reduction. *JAMA* 2004, 291(23):2821–2827.

[177] Berthold HK, Laaksonen R, Lehtimaki T, Gylling H, Krone W, Gouni-Berthold I: SREBP-1c gene polymorphism is associated with increased inhibition of cholesterol-absorption in response to ezetimibe treatment. *Exp Clin Endocrinol Diabetes* 2008, 116(5): 262–267.

[178] Perera V, Gross AS, McLachlan AJ: Influence of environmental and genetic factors on CYP1A2 activity in individuals of South Asian and European ancestry. *Clin Pharmacol Ther* 2012, 92(4):511–519.

[179] Willson MN, Neumiller JJ, Sclar DA, Robison LM, Skaer TL: Ethnicity/race, use of pharmacotherapy, scope of physician-ordered cholesterol screening, and provision of

diet/nutrition or exercise counseling during US office-based visits by patients with hyperlipidemia. *Am J Cardiovasc Drugs* 2010, 10(2):105–108.

[180] Billimek J, Malik S, Sorkin DH, Schmalbach P, Ngo-Metzger Q, Greenfield S, Kaplan SH: Understanding disparities in lipid management among patients with type 2 diabetes: gender differences in medication nonadherence after treatment intensification. *Women's Health Issues* 2015, 25(1):6–12.

[181] Hsia SH, Desnoyers ML, Lee ML: Differences in cholesterol management among states in relation to health insurance and race/ethnicity across the United States. *J Clin Lipidol* 2013, 7(6):675–682.

[182] Ratanawongsa N, Zikmund-Fisher BJ, Couper MP, Van Hoewyk J, Powe NR: Race, ethnicity, and shared decision making for hyperlipidemia and hypertension treatment: the DECISIONS survey. *Medical Decision Making* 2010, 30(5 Suppl):65S–76S.